CBS—Quick Medical Examination Review Series

ANAESTHESIA

FIFTEENTH EDITION

CBS—Quick Medical Examination Review Series

ANAESTHESIA

FIFTEENTH EDITION

Edited by :

DR. M.S. BHATIA (MD, Dip. WPA, MNAMS)
Professor & Head, Department of Psychiatry
University College of Medical Sciences
&
Guru Teg Bahadur Hospital,
Dilshad Garden, Delhi - 110095

Previously at :
Maulana Azad Medical College and Associated Hospitals, New Delhi
&
Lady Hardinge Medical College and Associated Hospitals, New Delhi

Contributing Editor :
DR. NIRMALJIT KAUR (MD)
Senior Specialist, Department of Microbiology
Dr. R.M.L. Hospital
New Delhi - 110001

Previously at :
LHMC & Smt. S.K. Hospital , New Delhi

CBS

CBS PUBLISHERS & DISTRIBUTORS PVT. LTD.
NEW DELHI • BANGALORE • PUNE • COCHIN • CHENNAI (INDIA)

DEDICATED TO
READERS WHO READ, UNDERSTAND
&
RECIPROCATE

ISBN : 978-81-239-1838-9

First Edition : 1992
Second Edition : 1993
Third Edition : 1994
Fourth Edition : 1995
Fifth Edition : 1996
Sixth Edition : 1997
Seventh Edition : 1998
Eighth Edition : 1999

Ninth Edition : 2000
Tenth Edition : 2001
Eleventh Edition : 2002
Twelveth Edition : 2003
Thirteenth Edition : 2004
Fourteenth Edition : 2005
Fifteenth Edition : 2010

Published by Satish Kumar Jain and produced by V.K. Jain for
CBS Publishers & Distributors Pvt. Ltd.,
CBS Plaza, 4819/XI Prahlad Street, 24 Ansari Road, Daryaganj,
New Delhi - 110002, India.
e-mail: cbspubs@vsnl.com, cbspubs@airtelmail.in, delhi@cbspd.com
Ph.: 23289259, 23266861, 23266867 • Fax: 011-23243014 • Website: www.cbspd.com

Branches:
• *Bangalore:* Seema House, 2975, 17th Cross, K.R. Road,
  Bansankari 2nd Stage, Bangalore - 560070
  Ph.: 26771678/79 • Fax: 080-26771680 • e-mail: bangalore@cbspd.com
• *Pune:* Shaan Brahmha Complex, 631/632, Basement, Appa Balwant Chowk,
  Budhwar Peth, Next to Ratan Talkies, Pune - 411002
  Ph.: 020-24464057/58 • Fax: 020-24464059 • e-mail: pune@cbspd.com
• *Cochin:* 36/14, Kalluvilakam, Lissie Hospital Road,
  Cochin - 682018, Kerala • e-mail: cochin@cbspd.com
  Ph.: 0484-4059061-65 • Fax: 0484-4059065
• *Chennai:* 20, West Park Road, Shenoy Nagar,
  Chennai - 600030 • e-mail: chennai@cbspd.com
  Ph.: 044-26260666-26202620 • Fax: 044-45530020

Printed at : Somya Printers, Delhi

PREFACE

Life is a continuous learning process. Human beings are born to learn and gain knowledge. Education is a means to acquire knowledge and skills that an individual desires to practise. Examinations are the means to evaluate the knowledge. Though no method of evaluation is without flaw, the process of standardization has resulted in a multiple choice system of examination. This system satisfies the basic qualities of a measuring instrument viz., validity, reliability and objectivity.

Recently, a number of books have been published about these examinations but the **best book still remains that which covers the maximum number of questions, which had been asked in that particular examination,** because the chance of repetition of these questions from so-called **"Question Bank"** remains very high. Recently, it has been observed that many **"Question Banks"** have overlapped. So, it is best to do a book which is complete and covers the **"Question Banks"** of maximum number of examinations. This book is being forwarded in this direction.

This book is designed as a supplement to the standard textbooks. It includes the **Referenced - MCQ's** (of previous years papers) of various PG Medical Entrance and Services Examinations **speciality-wise and Chapter-wise** arranged. The students while preparing the text or just before the examination can quickly go through this book. This will help in detecting the areas of weakness in understanding the text and thus, will improve the skills with multiple choice system of examination. It is a favourite book for **"Paper-setters"**.

The importance of doing MCQ's alongwith text has increased tremendously because, recently, it has become a tendency to frame MCQ's usually not covered by the standard textbooks followed at undergraduate level. **"Quick Medical Text Review Series"** can be a useful adjuant to this book.

Beware of the **Fraudulent Books** available in the market, which covers a part of copied **'Question Bank'** from this book, and also, based on **'Constructed'** rather than **'Original'** Question Book. It is suggested not to waste time on these books. Every MCQ matters a lot in a highly competitive exams.

I request the readers not to forget to send their opinions, as also suggestions and contributions if any, about all aspects of this book. It will be of invaluable help in enhancing the utility of the book in future.

All suggestions are welcome and will be duly acknowledged in future editions.

— **Editors**

A book of the Readers, for the
Readers, by the Readers

NOTE

The MCQ's of multiple response type (i.e. with **more than one correct answer** have been omitted in this Edition. Kindly refer to separate books **(PGI MD Entrance Exam & DNB Entrance Exam.** Part-I) by the same author and Publishers.

ADVICE

Read carefully the suggestions in the beginning of this book.

Prepare text from books suggested in the beginning and go through **Referenced MCQ's** of this book. Don't waste time in **inexperienced, incomplete and fraudulent courses books for PG Medical Entrance Examinations.**

ABOUT THE BOOK

This book has been compiled with the main aim to help the students to **quickly revise the Chapter-wise up-to-date referenced question** asked in various entrance examinations (Years indicated in the brackets).

Quick Medical Examinations Review Series contains Speciality-wise 45,000 MCQ's based on up-to-date papers from 1978 onwards.

The important examinations covered in this book (with code word in the bracket) are :

Examinations	Code used
(A) All India level	
1. All India Postgraduate Entrance Examination	(AI)
2. AIIMS MD Entrance Examination	(AIIMS)
3. PGI MD Entrance Examination	(PGI)
4. Combined Medical Services Examination by UPSC	(UPSC)
5. Civil Services Entrance Examination, Part-I (Medicine)	(CS)
6. Army Medical Corps Entrance Examination	(AMC)
7. Diplomate of National Board Entrance Examination	(DNB)
8. NIMHANS PG Entrance Examination	(NIMHANS)
9. Sanjay Gandhi PG Institute Entrance Examination	(SGPGI)
10. CIP Ranchi PG Entrance Examination	(CIP)
11. Manipal Academy of Higher Education PG Entrance Examination	(Manipal/MAHE)
12. Sree Chitra Tirunal Institute for Medical Science & Technology	(SCTIMST)
13. Command Hospital, Bangalore	(CH)
14. Bhabha Atomic Research Centre	(BARC)
15. Institute of Aerospace Medicine	(IAM)
(B) State level	
16. Delhi MD Entrance Examination	(Delhi)
17. Bihar MD Entrance Examination	(Bihar)
18. JIPMER PG Entrance Examination	(JIPMER)
19. CMC PG Entrance Examination	(CMC)
20. Rohtak PG Entrance Examination	(Rohtak)
21. MP State PG Entrance Examination	(MP)
22. AP State MD Entrance Examination	(AP)
23. TN State MD Entrance Examination	(TN)
24. Karnataka Postgraduate Medical Entrance Examination	(Karnataka)
25. Maharashtra PG Entrance Examination	(Maharashtra)
26. Kerala State MD Entrance Examination	(Kerala)
27. Rajasthan Postgraduate Entrance Examination	(Rajasthan)
28. PG Entrance Examination, Varanasi	(BHU)
29. Burdwan University	(BU)
30. Combined Entrance Examination for PG Courses, U.P.	(UP)
31. Punjab State PG Entrance Examination	(Punjab)
32. Aligarh Muslim University PG Entrance Examination	(AMU)
33. Nizam's Institute Entrance Examination, Hyderabad	(Nizam's)
34. Postgraduate Admission Test, Orissa	(Orissa)
35. Calcutta University Public Service Commission	(CUPSC)
36. TN Public Service Commission	(TNPSC)
37. Calcutta PG Entrance Examination	(Calcutta)
(C) Foreign	
PLAB, FCGP, GMC, FLEX, USMLE, MRCP, FRCS, MRCOG, etc.	

Sources of Errors (Anaesthesia)

Example 1 : **All are true about Glasgow coma scale except :** **AIIMS 1994, 99**
  A. Consists of eye opening, motor and verbal response
  B. Score is between 3-15
  C. Low Score indicates poor prognosis
  D. Obeying the motor command is given maximum score

Answer : None of the above (Harrison's 12th ed., pp. 2008) i.e. All the choices are correct.

Example 2 : **Following anaesthetic agent is hepatotoxic :** **AI 1988**
  A. Ether   B. Halothane
  C. Chloroform   D. Cyclopropane

Answer : Both (c) & (b) are correct

Example 3 : **Correct Composition of Sodalime is :** **Delhi 1993**
  NaOH   Ca(OH)2
  A. 5%   95%
  B. 15%   85%
  C. 20%   80%
  D. 80%   20%

Answer : None because the correct composition is 1% KOH, 4% NaOH and 95% Ca(OH)2

Example 4 : **For spinal anaesthesia, Bupivacaine is used in concentration (%) of :**
  Delhi 1993, 94
  A. 1   B. 2
  C. 4   D. 5

Answer : None of the above are true. Correct answer is 0.25-0.50%

Example 5 : **External cardiac message is given at the rate of :** **Delhi 1993, 95**
  A. 40/min   B. 60/min
  C. 80/min   D. 100/min
  Choice (b, c, d) Davidson's Principles and Practice of Medicine, 16th edition (Page 273)
  Choice (c) Harrison's Principles of Internal Medicine, 12th edition (Page 240)
  Choice (d) Miller's Textbook of Anaesthesia.

Advice
Questions with inaccurate language (structuring) or wrong choices should better be left unattempted.

IMPORTANT ANAESTHESIA TEXT FOR MCQ'S

Historical Aspects	History of General Anaesthesia (Discovery of N_2O, Ether, O_2, Chloroform, Cyclopropane, TCE, Halothane, Methoxyflurane), History of Local Anaesthesia (Spinal and epidural anaesthesia), Muscle Relaxants and Endotracheal intubation.
Premedications	Drugs used (Pentobarbital, Pethidine, Morphine, Promethazine, Atropine, Triclofos, Droperidol, Hyoscine), their doses, Adverse effects and Contraindications, Named formulae to estimate dose.
Local Anaesthesia	Techniques used, their Indications, Contraindications, Drugs used, (Lignocaine, Bupivacaine, Prilocaine, Cinchocaine), Subarachnoid and Extradural
General Anaesthesia	Theories and stages, Induction (Thiopentone, Methohexitone, Propanidid, Ketamine, Etomidate, Althesin, Suxamethonium, Scoline, d-TC), Agents (Ether, Halothane, N_2O, Cyclopropane, Methoxyflurane, Trilene, Chloroform, Enflurane, Isoflurane, Propofol, Fluorexene), Properties (colours & pressures of cylinders), Benefits, Drawbacks and contraindications, Maintenance (analgesics e.g. Fentanyl, Muscle relaxants e.g. Scoline, d-TC, Suxamethonium, Alcuronium, Pancuronium, Atracurium, Vecuronium).
Miscellaneous	Causes of difficult intubation, Common complications during anaesthesia (hypotension, arrythmias, pneumothorax, hypertension, vomiting, hypoventilation, intracranial pressure), Apparatus (Magill's circuits, Boyle's apparatus), I/V solutions, endotracheal tube size estimation), Important drug interactions, Anaesthesia in Special situations (Children/ Elderly/Pregnancy/Diabetes mellitus/Porphyria/Neuro or CVS surgery etc.), Important Physiological Factual data (Boiling temp. and partition coefficients of anaesthetics Respiratory, Liver and Kidney function tests etc.), Cardiopulmonary resuscitation.

IMPORTANT TIPS OF ANAESTHESIA

Read

*	Laws of physics related to anaesthesia	Lee's **Synopsis of Anaesthesia**
*	Induced arterial hypotension, indications & contraindications	Lee's **Synopsis of Anaesthesia**
*	Choice of anaesthetic agents in medical diseases	Lee's **Synopsis of Anaesthesia**
*	Surgical operations & choice of anaesthesia	Lee's **Synopsis of Anaesthesia**
*	Muscle relaxants in children	Lee's **Synopsis of Anaesthesia**
*	Comparison of Intravenous crystalloid fluids	Lee's **Synopsis of Anaesthesia**
*	About properties of Common anaesthetic agents	Table in Bhatia's **Quick Medical Text Review, Anaesthesia**
*	About History of anaesthetic agents	Bhatia's **Quick Medical Text Review, Anaesthesia**
*	About estimation of doses of intravenous anaesthetic agents	Bhatia's **Quick Medical Text Review, Anaesthesia**
*	About Thiopentone and other anaesthetic agents	Table in Bhatia's **Quick Medical Text Review, Anaesthesia**
*	About depolarizing Muscle relaxants	Lee's **Synopsis of Anaesthesia**
*	About preference of anaesthetic agents in various diseases	Bhatia's **Quick Medical Text Review, Anaesthesia**
*	About pressures in different gas cylinders and their colours	Table in Bhatia's **Quick Medical Text Review, Anaesthesia**
*	About causes of malignant hyperthermia	Lee's **Synopsis of Anaesthesia**
*	About extradural analgesia in obstetrics	Table in Bhatia's **Quick Medical Text Review, Anaesthesia**
*	About Physical properties of anaesthetic agents	Table in Bhatia's **Quick Medical Text Review, Anaesthesia**
*	About local anaesthetic agents	Table in Bhatia's **Quick Medical Text Review, Anaesthesia**
*	About Stages of anaesthesia	Tables in Bhatia's **Quick Medical Text Review, Anaesthesia**
*	One must read interactions of drugs and disease with anaesthetic agents and important points	Bhatia's **Quick Medical Text Review, Anaesthesia**
*	Important points & factual data	Bhatia's **Quick Medical Text Review, Anaesthesia**

CONTENTS

1

MCQ's OF HISTORICAL ASPECTS

What is important in Historical Aspects

History of General Anaesthesia (Discovery of N_2O, Ether, O_2, Chloroform, Cyclopropane, TCE, Halothane, Methoxyflurane), History of Local Anaesthesia (Spinal and Epidural Anaesthesia), Muscle Relaxants and Endotracheal intubation

1. The application of cocaine as local anaesthetic was first reported by : **AIIMS 1985, 89**
   A. Albert Niemann
   B. Sigmund Freud
   C. Karl Koller
   D. Joseph Brettauer

2. The first endotracheal intubation was done in 1880 without resorting to tracheostomy by :
   AIIMS 1985
   A. Sir Willaim Macewen
   B. Kirstein
   C. Chevalier Jackson
   D. Dorrance

3. Circulation of CSF was discovered in 1825 by :
   DNB 1993
   A. J.L. Corning
   B. H.I. Quincke
   C. F. Magendie
   D. G.E. Caglieri

4. Nitrous oxide with O2 was introduced by :
   AIIMS 1982
   A. Trendelenburg
   B. Priestley
   C. Davy
   D. Andrews

5. First reducing valve used in anaesthesia was designed by : **AIIMS 1982**
   A. Adam
   B. Heidbrink
   C. Endurance
   D. Beard
   E. Mckeeson

6. Oxygen was liberated by heating mercuric oxide in 1774 by : **AIIMS 1981**
   A. James Watt
   B. Joseph Priestley
   C. Humphary Davy
   D. Van Helmont

7. The analgesic properties of nitrous oxide was discovered by : **AIIMS 1982, 85**
   A. W.T.G Morton
   B. Humphry Davy
   C. Horace Wells
   D. Crawford W. Long

8. The credit of introducing successful nitrous oxide anaesthesia belongs to : **AIIMS 1982**
   A. Humphary Davy
   B. Horace Wells
   C. W.T.G. Morton
   D. John Snow

9. The first specialist in anaesthesia was :
   AIIMS 1982
   A. Benjamin Ward Richardson
   B. John Snow
   C. James Young Simpson
   D. Leopold

10. Who discovered IV anaesthesia : **PGI 1982**
    A. Johann Sigmund
    B. Humphry
    C. D.L. Tabern
    D. John S. Lundy

11. The word 'anaesthesia' was first used by :
    AIIMS 1984
    A. Oliver Wendell Holmes
    B. Horace Well
    C. W.T.G. Morton
    D. John Snow

12. The first public demonstration of Anaesthesia was done by : **JIPMER 1992**
    A. H.G. Wells
    B. John Snow
    C. I.W. Magill
    D. Thomas Green Morton

13. The Triad of anaesthesia are all of the following except : **JIPMER 1993, 95**
    A. Narcosis
    B. Analgesia
    C. Relaxation
    D. Amnesia

14. First Boyle Machine used for anaesthetic administration was produced in the year :
    Karnataka 1989
    A. 1890
    B. 1905
    C. 1917
    D. 1937

15. The first blind Nasal intubation was performed by :
    AIIMS 1982
    A. Rowbotham
    B. John Snow
    C. Macintosh
    D. Clover
    E. Robert Hooke

Ans.	1. C	2. A	3. C	4. D	5. D	6. B	7. B	8. C	9. B	10. D
	11. A	12. D	13. C	14. C	15. A					

16. The first physician Anaesthetist who realized that glass was not a good conductor of heat and cooling of ether lowered the inspired concentration of anaesthetic is :
    AIIMS 1983
    A. John Snow   B. Rowbotham
    C. Magill   D. Epstein and MacIntosh
    E. Goldman

17. The Concept of two different receptors alpha and beta, for catecholamine action was proposed by :
    AIIMS 1981
    A. Sir Henry Dale   B. Ahlquist
    C. King   D. Loewi
    E. Von Euler

18. The terminology, pH, was coined by :   **AIIMS 1983**
    A. Siggard-Anderson   B. Henderson-Hasselbach
    C. Sorenson   D. Davenport
    E. Astrup

19. Earliest local anaesthetic used was :   **AIIMS 1990**
    A. Lignocaine   B. Xylocaine
    C. Procainamide   D. Cocaine

20. Ether was discovered by :   **PGI 1986**
    A. Priestley   B. Snow
    C. Morton   D. Guedel
    E. Horace Wells

21. Guedel stages of anaesthesia was given for :
    Delhi 1988
    A. Ether   B. Halothane
    C. Cyclopropane   D. Trilene

22. Nitrous oxide was first introduced by :   **AMC 1982**
    A. Davy   B. Bernard
    C. Andrews   D. Wells
    E. Priestley

23. Inhalation/endotracheal anaesthesia in man was popularized by :   **AIIMS 1982**
    A. Mac Ewan   B. Snow
    C. Meltzer and Auer   D. Magill and Rowbotham
    E. None of the above

24. Ether was used for anaesthesia by :   **AIIMS 1994**
    A. Clarke   B. Cordis
    C. Jackson   D. Suckling

25. N_2O use began in :   **PGI 1995**
    A. 1850   B. 1856
    C. 1890   D. 1961

26. CSF was discovered in 1764 by :   **DNB 1994**
    A. William Harvey
    B. F. Magendie
    C. Domenico Cotugno
    D. Niemann and Lossen

27. First lumbar puncture was done by :   **UP 1998**
    A. Bier - 1861
    B. Jocoby Kiel - 1891
    C. Quincke - 1841
    D. Essex Wynter - 1860

28. In 1998, Nobel Prize was awarded for discovery of :
    AIIMS 1998
    A. Nitric oxide   B. Nitrous oxide
    C. Superoxide   D. H_2O_2

29. Intravenous Regional Anaesthesia was described by :
    Kerala 2000
    A. Macintosh   B. Magill
    C. Guedel   D. Bain
    E. Bier

Ans.	16. A	17. D	18. C	19. D	20. C	21. A	22. D	23. D	24. A	25. B
	26. C	27. C	28. C	29. E						

EXPLANATIONS OF HISTORICAL ASPECTS

1. Ans. — C. Karl Koller
2. Ans. — A. Sir Willaim Macewen
3. Ans. — C. F. Magendie
4. Ans. — D. Andrews

    Nitrous oxide gas was first prepared by Priestley (1733-1804) in 1772. Anaesthetic properties suggested by Sir Humphry Davy (1778-1829) in 1799. In 1808, P.C. Barton (1786 to 1808) of Philadelphia, again described the exhilarating effects of nitrous oxide. Edmund Andrews (1824-1904) of Chicago, combined it with oxygen to give longer anaesthesia. In 1878, Paul Bert (1830-1886) of France, administered it in a hyperbaric chamber.

5. Ans. — D. Beard
6. Ans. — B. Joseph Priestley
7. Ans. — B. Humphry Davy
8. Ans. — C. W.T.G. Morton
9. Ans. — B. John Snow
10. Ans. — D. John S. Lundy
11. Ans. — A. Oliver Wendell Holmes
12. Ans. — D. Thomas Green Morton

    W.T.G. Morton of Boston in the U.S. gave ether at the Massachusetts General Hospital on 16th October 1846 to Gilbert Abbott.

13. Ans. — C. Relaxation
14. Ans. — C. 1917
15. Ans. — A. Rowbotham
16. Ans. — A. John Snow
17. Ans. — D. Loewi
18. Ans. — C. Sorenson
19. Ans. — D. Cocaine
20. Ans. — C. Morton

    William Thomas Green Morton deserves the chief credit for introduction of ether as an anaesthetic agent, although W.E. Clarke (1818-1878) of Rochester, New York gave ether for a dental extraction in 1842).

21. Ans. — A. Ether
22. Ans. — D. Wells
23. Ans. — D. Magill and Rowbotham
24. Ans. — A. Clarke
25. Ans. — B. 1856
26. Ans. — C. Domenico Cotugno
27. Ans. — C. Quincke - 1841
28. Ans. — C. Superoxide
29. Ans. — E. Bier

2

IMPORTANT TEXT OF PREMEDICATION

PREMEDICATION OF CHOICE

		Males	Females	Children
Neonate - 2 years	Atropine S/C or I/M			
Preterm	0.1 mg			
upto 10 kg	0.2 mg			
10-20 kg	0.4 mg			
> 20 kg	0.6 mg			
2-8 years	Trimeprazine tartarate orall Phenothiazine)			
	2-4 mg/kg (1-2 mg/lb) 0.6 - 1.2 mg atropine			
8-65 years	Papaveretum	20 mg	15 mg	2 mg/6kg
	Hyoscine	0.4	0.3 mg	
	Pethidine	100 mg	75 mg	10 mg/6kg
65-70 years	Narcotics + Atropine			
> 70 years	only atropine			

PARTIAL LIST OF METHODS USED FOR ESTIMATING DOSES FOR INFANTS AND CHILDREN OF HISTORICAL INTEREST

Gaubius Method :

Children under 1 year receive 1/12 adult dose.

Children under 2 years receive 1/8 adult dose.

Children under 4 years receive 1/4 adult dose.

Children under 20 receive 2/3 adult dose

Brunton's Rule

$$\frac{Age}{25} \times adult\ dose.$$

Cowling's Rule :

$$\frac{Age + 1}{24} \times adult\ dose$$

Dilling's Rule :

$$\frac{Age}{Age + 12} \times adult\ dose$$

Fried Rule :

$$\frac{Age\ in\ months}{150} \times adult\ dose$$

Clark's Rule :

$$\frac{Weight\ of\ pt.\ in\ lb}{150} \times adult\ dose$$

(Contd...)

PARTIAL LIST OF METHODS USED FOR ESTIMATING DOSES FOR INFANTS AND CHILDREN OF HISTORICAL INTEREST (Contd....)

Clark's Surface Area Rule :

$$\frac{\text{Surface area child}}{\text{Surface area adult}} \times \text{adult dose}$$

Augsburger's Rule :

(Wt. in kg x 1.5) + 10 = % of adult dose

or (Age x 4) + 20 = % of adult dose.

Cullis's Rule :

$$\frac{\text{Wt. of child in 1b}}{100} \times \text{adult dose.}$$

This rule aims to compensate for the low doses estimated by Clark's rule for infants and small children.

Allometric Law of Differential Growth : (Sticker G.B. 1964)

Y = a + X where Y = drug dose

a and b = constants

X = weight in kg.

Doses may also be expressed in terms of mg per kg. Different quantities per unit of body weight are usually described for small infants, larger infants and children, and for adults (the surface area rule requires only one set of terms for all ages, i.e. mg/m2).

Churchill (1964) proposes relaxing all rules by the `mushroom eaters method' *provided that the disease affords one the luxury of time.*

Lastly, one cannot resist quoting Edward W. Pelikan's peculiar proposals:

Pelikan's Rule No. 1 :   Count the total number of deciduous and permanent teeth that have erupted, express the count as a fraction of the adult complement of 52 (20 + 32) and administer that fraction of the adult dose.

Pelikan's Rule No. 2 :   Paediatric dose = Body weight in kg x 7/8 = Percent of adult dose.

DRUGS USED FOR PREMEDICATION

Opioid analgesics	Benzodiazepines	Butyrophenones	Phenothiazines	Anticholinergics	Antiemetics
Morphine	Diazepam	Haloperidol	Promethazine	Atropine	Metoclopramide
Papaveretum	Nitrazepam	Droperidol	Promazine	Hyoscine	Butyrophenones
Pethidine	Flurazepam		Trimeprazine	Glycopyrolate	Phenothiazines
Phenoperidine	Lorazepam		Chlorpromazine		
Fentanyl	Flunitrazepam				
Pentazocine	Temazepam				
Buprenorphine					

MCQ's OF PREMEDICATIONS

What is important in Premedications

Drugs used (Pentobarbital, Pethidine, Morphine, Promethazine, Atropine, Triclofos, Droperidol, Hyoscine), their doses, Adverse effects and Contraindications, Named formulae to estimate dose

1. **Flushing of the face is more commonly encountered in children following premedication with except:**
   AIIMS 1988, 90
   A. Promethazine
   B. Atropine
   C. Diazepam
   D. Glycopyrolate

2. **Minimum respiratory depression is caused by:**
   AIIMS 1986, 87, 91
   A. Morphine
   B. Pethidine
   C. Fentanyl
   D. Pentazocine

3. **The most preferred drug for induction is :**
   Kerala 1996
   A. Thiopentone
   B. Etomidate
   C. Fentanyl
   D. Ketamine

4. **The dose of trimeparazine (an antihistaminic used for premedication for anaesthesia) is :** **AIIMS 1985**

	Oral dose (mg/kg)	I/M dose (mg/kg)
A.	1—2	0.5
B.	2—4	1.0
C.	4—6	2.0
D.	6—8	3.0

5. **Local constriction is seen with :** **AIIMS 1997**
   A. Cocaine
   B. Xylocaine
   C. Bupivacaine
   D. Mivacaine

6. **Epinephrine is contraindicated in following except :**
   AIIMS 1997
   A. Hypertension
   B. Thyrotoxicosis
   C. Bronchial asthma
   D. Pheochromocytoma

7. **Bronchospasm is caused by all except :**
   PGI 1988, 89
   A. Morphine
   B. Halothane
   C. Ether
   D. Nitrous oxide

8. **Pethidine is not given with :** **Delhi 1985, 86**
   A. Pentazocine
   B. Beta blockers
   C. MAO inhibitors
   D. Alpha blockers

9. **Recommended dosage of morphine for premedication of a 7 lb infant is about :** **AIIMS 1984**
   A. 0.5 mg
   B. 0.7 mg
   C. 0.9 mg
   D. 1.0 mg
   E. None of the above

10. **Fentanyl is contraindicated in all except :**
    AMU 1987
    A. Liver failure
    B. Kidney failure
    C. Head injury
    D. MAOI therapy

11. **Post-operative restlessness is seen in induction with :**
    Delhi 1986
    A. Narcotic premedication
    B. Barbiturate premedication
    C. Full badder
    D. Anoxia

12. **Which of the following is used as pre-analsthetic medication causes longest amnesia :** **MP 1998**
    A. Diazepam
    B. Lorezapam
    C. Midazolam
    D. Flunitrezepam

13. **Color of thiopentone is :** **Delhi 1996**
    A. Blue
    B. Orange
    C. White
    D. Colourless

14. **Subarachnoid space is :** **Delhi 1996**
    A. T10-11
    B. T11-12
    C. S1, 2
    D. S2, 3

15. **Number of type of receptors for morphine is :**
    PGI 1993
    A. 2
    B. 4
    C. 6
    D. 8

16. **Narcotic antagonist/s free from agonist activity is/are:**
    AP 1990, 91, 94
    A. Naloxone
    B. Nalorphine
    C. Levallorphan
    D. Only B and C are true
    E. All of the above

Ans.	1. B	2. D	3. A	4. B	5. A	6. C	7. C	8. C	9. E	10. D
	11. B	12. D	13. D	14. D	15. C	16. A				

17. When neonatal respiratory depression occur, Narcotic Antagonist should be given to: Bihar 1991
    A. Mother before delivery
    B. Baby umbilical vein after birth
    C. Both mother and baby after delivery
    D. Only mother after delivery
    E. None of the above

18. Diazepam toxicity can be specifically antagonized by: JIPMER 1992
    A. Neooctinum   B. Naloxone
    C. Doxapram   D. Flumazenil

19. Correct placement of endotracheal tube can be judged by following except :   Rajasthan 1996
    A. Bilateral breath sounds over lungs
    B. Chest X-ray
    C. Increased heart rate & fever
    D. Arterial CO2 measurement

20. Pre-operative (abdominal) duration for which a patient must be advised to avoid smoking: TN 1990
    A. One week   B. Two weeks
    C. Three weeks   D. None of the above

21. The anaesthetist is using atropine should remember :   AIIMS 1984
    A. Tachycardia is produced
    B. Sweating is increased
    C. Hypothermia is produced
    D. Metabolic depression causes decreased oxygen requirement

22. The aims of premedication are the following except: AIIMS 1985; UPSC 1987; Rohtak 2001
    A. Reduction of apprehension
    B. Drying of secretions
    C. Production of amnesia
    D. Increase in protective reflex activity
    E. Potentiation of anaesthetic effects of anaesthetic agents

23. Effect of atropine as pre-anaesthetic agent include all of the following except: AIIMS 1982
    A. It reduces salivation
    B. It raises body temperature
    C. It reduces vagal effect on heart
    D. It induces sleep
    E. It reduces bronchial secretions

24. Which of the following is not present in acute morphine poisoning :   AIIMS 1983
    A. Decreased urinary output
    B. Hyperpyrexia
    C. Slow respiration
    D. Pinpoint pupil

25. All except following may be used for premedication: AIIMS 1984
    A. Diazepam   B. Papaverine
    C. Atropine   D. Pancuronium

26. A female patient in the first trimester of pregnancy requires surgery. Which of the following drugs is the least desirable pre-operative medication or maintenance agent :   DNB 1991
    A. Morphine   B. Meperidine
    C. Glycopyrolate   D. Diazepam
    E. Pancuronium

27. Which of the following is not a contraindication for use of morphine :   AMU 1986
    A. Old age   B. Bronchial asthma
    C. Head injury   D. Renal colic

28. Morphine depresses: AP 1990
    A. Brain stem
    B. Spinal cord
    C. Cerebral cortex
    D. All levels of neuro axis

29. Dose of atropine per kg body weight is: Delhi 1989
    A. 10 mg   B. 0.1 mg
    C. 0.01 mg   D. 0.001 mg

30. Antisialagogue is the drug which: DNB 1989
    A. Increases heart rate
    B. Increase intestinal motility
    C. Decreases respiration
    D. Decreases the secretion of GI tract

31. Which of the following drugs is best suited for out patient anaesthesia :   AIIMS 1994
    A. Morphine   B. Pethidine
    C. Fentanyl   D. Alfentanyl

32. Dose of Thiopentone sodium for inducing anaesthesia is :   Orissa 1998
    A. 1-2 mg/kg   B. 4-7 mg/kg
    C. 8-10 mg/kg   D. 12-14 mg/kg

33. Which intravenous induction agent is preferred most :   Orissa 1999
    A. Thiopentone   B. Diazepam
    C. Ketamine   D. Methomine

34. About thiopentone, all are true except :   Kerala 1999
    A. Fast recovery
    B. Tendency to cause post-operative discomfort
    C. Causes laryngospasm
    D. Stage of delirium absent

Ans.	17. B	18. D	19. C	20. D	21. A	22. D	23. D	24. B	25. D	26. D
	27. D	28. D	29. C	30. D	31. D	32. B	33. A	34. D		

35. A 30-years old woman is to have a caesarean section under subdural anaesthesia with hyperbaric lignocaine. The management would include all the following except :   **UPSC 2000**
   A. "Preloading" her with a litre of saline
   B. Pre-medicating her with pethidine
   C. Putting a wedge under her right buttock after the block
   D. Atropine administration

36. Which of the following orders of speed of recovery and return of psychomotor function is correct :   **TNPSC 1998**
   A. Thiopentone>midazolam>propofol>methohexitone
   B. Midazolam>methohexitone>propofol>thiopentone
   C. Methohexitone>propofol>midazolam>thiopentone
   D. Propofol>methohexitone>thiopentone>midazolam

37. Following are used in pre-anaesthetic agent except :   **UP 2000**
   A. Morphine   B. Hyosine
   C. Neostigmine   D. Scopolamine

38. A 5 years old boy suffering from Duchenne muscular dystrophy and polymyositis has been fasting for 8 hours and has to undergo tendon lengthening procedure, which anaesthetics should be used :   **AIIMS 2000**
   A. Induction by I.V. thiopentone & N_2O & halothane for maintenance.
   B. Induction by I.V. propofol, N_2O & O2 for maintenance.
   C. Induction by I.V. scolone, and N_2O halothane for maintenance.
   D. Inhalational N_2O, halothane and oxygen for maintenance.

39. Which one of the following is not effective in abolishing post-anaesthetic shivering that is not related to hypothermia :   **Kerala 2000**
   A. Pethidine   B. Morphine
   C. Butorphanol   D. Tramadol
   E. Buprenorphine

40. Drug causing anaphylactic reaction :   **PGI 1998**
   A. Propofol   B. Alcuronium
   C. Thiopentone   D. Glycopyrolate

41. Safe inducing agent in malignant hyperpyrexia is :   **Delhi 2001**
   A. Thiopentone   B. Etomidate
   C. Halothane   D. Propofol

42. Pulse oximeter works on the following principle :   **COMEDK 2005**
   A. Beer Lambert's law
   B. Raman scattering effect
   C. Venturi principle
   D. Mass pectometry

Ans.	35. D	36. A	37. C	38. B	39. D	40. B	41. D	42. A

EXPLANATIONS OF PREMEDICATIONS

1.   Ans.— B.   Atropine

2.   Ans.— D.   Pentazocine

3.   Ans.— A.   Thiopentone

4.   Ans.— B.   2—4   1.0

5.   Ans.— A.   Cocaine

6.   Ans.— C.   Bronchial asthma

7.   Ans.— C.   Ether

8.   Ans.— C.   MAO inhibitors

> Pethidine in patients under MAOI causes alarming reactions (restlessness, hypertension, convulsions and coma- sometimes reversed by acidifying the urine) with absent tendon jerks and an extensor response; hypotension. The reaction is due to interference with microsomes in liver cells which detoxicate pethidine.

9.   Ans.— E.   None of the above

10.   Ans.— D.   MAOI therapy

11.   Ans.— B.   Barbiturate premedication

12.   Ans.— D.   Flunitrezepam

13.   Ans.— D.   Colourless

14.   Ans.— D.   S2, 3

15.   Ans.— C.   6

16.   Ans.— A.   Naloxone

> Naloxone is n-allyl nor oxymorphane and is derived from potent oxymorphone. It was synthesized in 1972. It antogonises the respiratory depression caused by pentazocine and dextropropoxyphene. It relaxes spasm of sphincter oddi. Duration of action is 1 hour. Naloxone unlike other drugs, has no intrinsic agonist activity. Its half life is 20 min and is metabolised in liver. Dose is 0.1-0.4 mg I/V repeated. In neonates 0.01 mg/kg.

17.   Ans.— B.   Baby umbilical vein after birth

> Pentazocine is used at the end of operation to reverse the respiratory depressant effects of fentanyl, while at the same time giving prolonged post-operative analgesia- 'sequential anaesthesia'.

18.   Ans.— D.   Flumazenil

19.   Ans.— C.   Increased heart rate & fever

20.   Ans.— D.   None of the above

21.   Ans.— A.   Tachycardia is produced

> It is due to vagolytic action.

22.   Ans.— D.   Increase in protective reflex activity

23.   Ans.— D.   It induces sleep

24.   Ans.— B.   Hyperpyrexia

> Morphine and related opiods produce respiratory depression, nausea, vomiting, dizziness, mental clouding, dysphoria, pruritus, constipation, increased pressure in biliary tract, urinary, retention and hypotension. Morphine is a direct metabolic depressant. Morphine was first isolated from opium by FWA Serturner (1783-1841). Chemial structure was determined in 1925 and was synthesized by Gates and Tschudi (1952).

25.   Ans.— D.   Pancuronium

26.   Ans.— D.   Diazepam

27.   Ans.— D.   Renal colic

28.   Ans.— D.   All levels of neuro axis

29.   Ans.— C.   0.01 mg

30.   Ans.— D.   Decreases the secretion of GI tract

> Atropine and Hyoscine are examples.

31.   Ans.— D.   Alfentanyl

32.   Ans.— B.   4-7 mg/kg

33.   Ans.— A.   Thiopentone

34.   Ans.— D.   Stage of delirium absent

35. Ans. — D. Atropine administration

36. Ans. — A. Thiopentone > midazolam > propofol > methohexitone

37. Ans. — C. Neostigmine

Neostigmine was isolated in 1804 from Calabar bean by Sir. T.R. Fraser. Anticurare action was discovered by Jacob Pal (1863-1936) in 1900. It is used to counter effects of d-tubocurare. Dose is 2.5 mg repeated carefully upto a total of 5 mg with atropine 1.5 mg or glyco-pyrronium.

38. Ans. — B. Induction by I.V. propofol, N_2O & O2 for maintenance.

39. Ans. — D. Tramadol

40. Ans. — B. Alcuronium

41. Ans. — D. Propofol

42. Ans. — A. Beer Lambert's law

3

IMPORTANT TEXT OF LOCAL ANAESTHESIA

LOCAL ANAESTHETIC TECHNIQUES

Indications

1. Any procedure for which local anaesthesia will provide satisfactory operating conditions.
2. Pulmonary disease provided that the patient will be able to tolerate required for the operation.
3. Previous adverse reaction to general anaesthetic agents.
4. Anticipated problems with maintaining the airways or intubation.
5. Urgent operation without adequate starvation. If time is available, it is preferable to starve the patient when large doses of local anaesthetic are to be used because a toxic reaction may cause depression of laryngeal reflexes, hypotension and vomiting.

Absolute contraindications

1. Refusal by the patient.
2. Allergy to local anaesthetic drugs.
3. Infection at the site of injection.
4. Anticoagulant therapy.
5. Bleeding diathesis.
6. Use of adrenaline - Containing solutions for patients on tricyclic antidepressants. Felypressin containing solutions are safe for these patients.

Relative Contraindications

1. Lack of patient cooperation.
2. Neurological disease - An exacerbation may be blamed on the anaesthetic technique.

Local anaesthetic toxicity

Prevention

1. Never exceed the maximum dose

	Plain	*With adrenaline*
Bupivacaine	2 mg/kg 4-hourly	2 mg/kg 4-hourly
Lignocaine	3 mg/kg	7 mg/kg
Prilocaine	6 mg/kg	8.5 mg/kg

NB: 1 ml of 1% solution contains 10 mg

The maximum dose of adrenaline is 500 mg- i.e. o.5 ml 1 : 1000 solution. The concentration of adrenaline should never exceed 1 : 200000. To achieve a concentration of 1 : 250000 put 4 drops of 1 : 1000 adrenaline through a 21 gauge needle into 25 ml anaesthetic solution.

2. Use the lowest dose and concentration of local anaesthetic which will provide satisfactory operating conditions.
3. Inject local anaesthetic slowly and aspirate frequently.
4. Use reduced doses in elderly and debilitated frequently.

Signs of toxicity

Central nervous system

Nervousness, tremor and convulsions are followed by respiratory depression and apnea.

Cardiovascular system

Severe hypotension may be followed by cardiac arrest.

Gastrointestinal system

There may be nausea, vomiting and abdominal pain.

Allergy

A rash, bronchospasm or anaphylactic shock may occur.

Treatment of a toxic reaction

Respiratory depression

Maintain the airway, intubating if necessary, give 100% oxygen and assist or control ventilation.

Convulsions

Give diazepam 0.1-0.2 mg/kg slowly IV

      or paraldehyde 10 ml IM

      or thiopentone 1-2 mg/kg IV slowly plus suxamethonium 1 mg/kg IV.

Then intubate and ventilate, remembering to take precautions if the stomach is not empty.

Hypotension

Give oxygen via a face mask even if respiratory is satisfactory, elevate the legs and give up to 1 litre of human plasma protein fraction, dextran 70 or Haemaccel, if the blood pressure does not rise give ephedrine 15-30 mg IM or metaraminol 1-2 mg IV.

Premedication

The choice depends on the anaesthesia personal preference.

Some suggestions are:

1.   Diazepam 10-20 mg orally 1 hour pre-operatively.
2.   Lorazepam 2-4 mg orally 1 hour pre-operatively.
3.   Papaveretum 10-20 mg plus droperidol 5-10 mg IM 1 hour pre-operatively.

These may be supplemented during the operation by a mixture of fentanyl 0.1 mg plus droperidol 10 mg made upto 5 ml with water. Give 1 ml increments IV, watching for sedation and signs of overdose (i.e. respiratory depression or hypotension).

DIFFERENCES BETWEEN SUBARACHNOID AND EXTRADURAL BLOCK

	SAB	Extradural
Dose of drug employed	Small. The drug has no action other than within the spinal cord	Large Systemic absorption occurs with possible CNS effects (drowsiness or fits) and cardiovascular effects (myocardial depression and peripheral dilatation).
Rate of onset of action	Fast—2.8 min	Slow : 20-40 min
Site of action	On spinal cord and spinal nerve roots	Various 1. Diffusions across dura into c.s.f. 2. Diffusion into c.s.f. via spinal nerve root dural cuffs. 3. Paravertebral nerve blocks

(Contd...)

DIFFERENCES BETWEEN SUBARACHNOID AND EXTRADURAL BLOCK (Contd..)

	SAB	Extradural
Success rate	100% if lumbar puncture successful	Missed segments, total failure not uncommon
Extent of block	May be extensive—dependent on positioning	Dependent on dose injected (rather than volume) Position of patient has small effect.
Intensity of block	May be complete	Rarely complete block of all nerve pathways
Segmental block	No	Yes
Addition of vasoconstrictor	Prolongs block in lumbar and sacral segments. With lignocaine and bupivacaine amethocaine block is prolonged reliably with phenylephrine but not with adrenaline.	Prolongs block with lignocaine. No significant effect with bupivacaine.

FACTORS INFLUENCING SPREAD OF HYPERBARIC SPINAL SOLUTIONS

Factors	Effects
Position of patient	Sitting position produces perineal block. In lateral position, block more pronounced on dependent side.
Spinal curvature	Because of lumbar lordosis, solutions may spread up to T 4 with patient horizontal and supine.
Speed of injection	Rapid injections cause dilution with c.s.f. thereby reducing the effect of gravity. Produces a higher level of block but may be less intense.
Barbotage	Dilutes the local anaesthetic, increase the height of block but may reduce the intensity. Vigerous barbotage may produce a solution too weak to produce any block.
Interspace chosen	Higher the interspace, higher the block.
Dose of drug	The larger the dose and concentration, the more intense the block and the longer the duration.
Sp.gr. of drug	Hyperbaric solutions move under the influences of gravity.
Fixation	The concentration of local anaesthetic decreases below a blocking concentration after 15-20 min. Subsequent alteration in patient's position does not cause further spread of block.

EXTRADURAL ANALGESIA IN OBSTETRICS

Indications	Contraindications
Pain and maternal request	*Absolute*
Incoordinate uterine contraction	Local sepsis
Pre-eclampia	Anatomical deformity
Premature labour	Ongoing neurological disease
Cardiovascular disease	Bleeding tendency
Diabetes mellitus	Anticoagulant therapy
Multiple pregnancy	Hypovolemia
Breech presentation	*Relative*
Forceps delivery	Previous LSCS
Caesarean section	Abruptio placentae

FEATURES OF INDIVIDUAL LOCAL ANAESTHETICS

Proper name	Conc.	Duration	Toxicity	pK	Partition Coeff.	% Protein bound	Main use
Cocaine	1	0.50	V. high	8.7	?	?	Nil
Benzocaine	N/A	2	Low	2.9	?	?	Topical
Procaine	2	0.75	Low	8.9	0.6	5.8	Nil
Chloroprocaine	1	0.75	Low	9.1	1	?	Not available
Amethocaine	0.25	2	High	8.5	80	76	Topical
Lignocaine	1	1	Medium	7.7	3	64	Infiltration Nerve block Extradural
Mepivacaine	1	1	Medium	7.6	1	77	Not available
Prilocaine	1	1.50	Low	7.7	1	55	Infiltration Nerve block IVRA
Cinchocaine	0.25	2	High	7.9	?	?	Spinal
Bupivacine	0.25	2-4	Medium	8.1	28	95	Extradural Spinal nerve block
Etidocaine	0.5	2-4	Medium	7.7	141	94	Not available

* Lignocaine = 1; N/A = Not applicable—not used in solution.
? = information not available.
NB. All figures are approximations as there is some variation in published values.

USE OF LIGNOCAINE AS LOCAL ANAESTHETIC

Anaesthesia	%
Skin infilteration	0.5 %
I.V. Regional	0.5 %
Minor nerve block	1.0 %
Brachial plexus	1.0 - 1.5 %
Sciatic/ femoral	1.0 - 1.5 %
Extradural	1.5 - 2.0 %
Spinal	2.0 - 5.0 %
Tonometry	4.0 %

MCQ's OF LOCAL ANAESTHESIA

What is important in Local Anaesthesia

Techniques used, their Indications, Contraindications, Drugs used, Lignocaine, Bupivacaine, Prilocaine, Cinchocaine), Subarachnoid and Extradural

1. Concerning Cauda equina syndrome, characteristic features include all of the following except :
   AIIMS 1984, 96
   A. Incontinence of faeces
   B. Retention of urine
   C. Loss of sexual function
   D. Incontinence of urine

2. Local analgesic drugs preferred for its use in dentistry is : **AIIMS 1988, 92**
   A. Etiodocaine   B. Prilocaine
   C. Bupivacaine   D. Amethocaine

3. LA induced arrhythmia is treated with :
   Rajasthan 1998, 2000
   A. Bretylium   B. Phenytoin
   C. Verapamil   D. Lignocaine

4. Cranial nerves not involved in spinal anaesthesia :
   AMC 1985; PGI 1987
   A. 1st and 10th   B. 3rd and 6th
   C. 2nd and 4th   D. 7th and 8th

5. A local anaesthetic which is ineffective topically is :
   Kerala 1989
   A. Lidocaine   B. Tetracaine
   C. Mepivacaine   D. Cocaine

6. Spinal anaesthesia is preferred in lower abdominal surgeries because it : **AIIMS 1987**
   A. Gives deep analgesia
   B. Gives good relaxation of abdominal muscles.
   C. Shrinks intestines so that other viscera are seen well.
   D. Patients is conscious and co-operative.

7. The duration of effect of spinal anaesthesia depends upon : **AIIMS 1986**
   A. The site of injection
   B. Quantity of drug injected
   C. Type of drug used
   D. All the above

8. The following effects are seen after spinal anaesthesia except : **AIIMS 1985**
   A. Respiratory paralysis
   B. Decrease in arterial blood pressure
   C. Nausea and vomiting
   D. Different nerve block

9. The following are true except : **DNB 1989**
   A. The epidural space is between the dura and the bony and ligamentous walls of spinal canal.
   B. Large doses of local anaesthetic are required to produce epidural anaesthesia.
   C. The onset of sympathetic block is slower than in spinal.
   D. Fall in blood pressure in epidural block is more when compared to spinal block.

10. Epidural block is indicated in all except :
    DNB 1989
    A. Patients in hypovolemia
    B. Patients with asthma and bronchitis
    C. Post-operative pain relief
    D. Obstetric analgesia

11. Addition of Adrenaline with local anaesthetic during spinal subarachnoid block may cause :
    Bihar 1990
    A. Demyelination of nerves
    B. Anterior spinal artery syndrome
    C. Acute mellitus
    D. None of the above

12. Application of cold to a localized part of the body to block local nerve conduction of painful stimuli is known as : **AMC 1982**
    A. Cryotherapy
    B. Refrigeration Analgesia
    C. Induced Hypothermia
    D. Acupuncture
    E. Cardio pulmonary Bypass

Ans.	1. D	2. B	3. A	4. A	5. A	6. C	7. C	8. A	9. D	10. A
	11. B	12. B								

13. The effects of chilling in refrigeration analgesia includes :   **AIIMS 1982**
A. Interference with Conduction of nerve impulse
B. Reduction of metabolic rate and oxygen requirement
C. Inhibition of bacterial growth and infection
D. Retardation of healing
E. All of the above

14. Shortest acting depolarizing agent is :
                                        Rajasthan 1998
A. Alcuronium   B. Gallamine
C. Mivacurlium   D. Pancuronium

15. Concerning Barbotage :   **AIIMS 1984**
A. Fluid (spinal) is alternately withdrawn and reinjected under pressure.
B. Technique used Epidural Analgesia.
C. Technique popularized in caudal Analgesia.
D. Cannot be carried out under hypothermic conditon.

16. Technique using solutions of local Anaesthetic drug with a higher specific gravity than of CSF is :
                                        AIIMS 1986
A. Hypobaric   B. Barbotage
C. Hypotensive   D. Hyperbaric
E. None of the above

17. During epidural anagesia the following points suggest that needle is in the extradural space :   **AIIMS 1983**
A. Loss of resistance sign
B. Negative pressure sign
C. Macintosh Extradural space indicator
D. All of the above
E. Only A and C is true

18. Needle used for epidural analgesia is are :
                                        AIIMS 1983
A. Straight Wide Bore 16-18 SWG needle
B. Huber point Tuohy needle
C. Straight fine bore 24 SWG needle
D. A and B are true
E. A and C are true

19. Theories of causation of Post spinal headache include all of the following except :   **Rohtak 1989**
A. Low CSF pressure
B. Normal CSF pressure
C. Aseptic Meningeal reaction
D. Both 'C and D' due to high CSF pressure

20. Treatment of spinal headache is :
                            Delhi 1984; Bihar 1990
A. IV fluids with head end of bed elevated.
B. Make the patient sit up and reduce fluid intake.
C. Large quantitiy of IV fluids with foot end of bed elevated.
D. Strict bed rest with IV lasix.

21. Following are true about I/V lignocaine except :
                                        Delhi 1993
A. Used in treatment of cardiac arrhythmias
B. Does not cross blood brain barrier
C. May cause vosoconstriction
D. Undergoes metabolism in liver

22. For inducing spinal anaesthesia the drug (local anaesthetic) is injected into :   **Delhi 1984**
A. Spinal cord   B. Subdural space
C. Subarachnoid space   D. Extradural space

23. For giving epidural block, the local anaesthesia is injected into :   **Delhi 1987**
A. Spinal cord   B. Subdural space
C. Subarachnoid space   D. Extradural space

24. Local anaesthetic for inducing spinal anaesthesia is injected into space between :   **Delhi 1983**
A. L1-L2 vertebrae   B. D12-L1 vertebrae
C. L3-L4 vertebrae   D. L5-S1 vertebrae

25. All are true for bupivacaine except :   **DNB 1990**
A. Long acting
B. Action is prolonged by addition of adrenaline
C. Maximum safe dose is 200 mg
D. Solutions can be autoclaved

26. Methaemoglobinaemia is seen due to one of the following local analgesic drug :
                                        Karnataka 1990
A. Procaine   B. Lignocaine
C. Prilocaine   D. Bupivacaine
E. Etidocaine

27. Longer lasting action is due to one of the following local analgesic drug :   **AMU 1987**
A. Lignocaine   B. Etidocaine
C. Bupivocaine   D. Prilocaine
E. Cocaine

28. Epidural narcotic is preferred over epidural LA because it causes :   **AIIMS 1990**
A. Less respiratory depression
B. No causes retention of urine
C. No motor paralysis
D. Less dose required

29. The following is not used when giving local anaesthesia in the fingers :   **AP 1990**
A. 2% Xylocaine   B. Rubber tourniquet
C. Ring block   D. Adrenaline

Ans.	13. E	14. C	15. A	16. D	17. D	18. D	19. B	20. C	21. B	22. B
	23. D	24. C	25. D	26. C	27. C	28. C	29. D			

30. **An increased dose of spinal anaesthetic is indicated in a patient who :** PGI 1981
    A. Is old
    B. Is pregnant
    C. Is obese
    D. Has ascites
    E. Has an abdominal tumour

31. **The advantage of epidural anaesthesia over spinal anaesthesia include :** AIIMS 1982
    A. Prolonged post-operative analgesia
    B. No post-operative headache
    C. Less chances of meningeal infection
    D. All of the above

32. **Complications of spinal anaesthesia include :** AIIMS 1984
    A. Headache
    B. Diplopia
    C. Cauda equina syndrome
    D. Retention of urine
    E. All of the above

33. **Which of the following affects dosage of spinal anaesthesia :** AMU 1989
    A. Height of the patient
    B. Obesity of the patient
    C. Pregnancy
    D. Ascites
    E. None of the above

34. **Average time for persistence of post-spinal headache is :** AMU 1990
    A. 4 hours
    B. 24 hours
    C. 3-4 days
    D. 3-4 weeks

35. **Spinal headache usually occurs on :** DNB 1991
    A. 1st post-operative day
    B. 2nd post-operative day
    C. 4th post-operative day
    D. 7th post-operative day

36. **Which of the following is most common sequela (though rare) of spinal anaesthesia :** DNB 1990
    A. Transverse myelitis
    B. Meningomyelitis
    C. Ascending myelitis
    D. Cauda equina syndrome

37. **In spinal anaesthesia, the last fibres to be blocked are those of :** AIIMS 1984; Delhi 1985; WB 1998
    A. Temperature
    B. Pain
    C. Pressure
    D. Motor and proprioceptive in high concentration

38. **Regarding post-spinal headache :** AIIMS 1984
    A. It has occipital and nuchal components.
    B. Never present during operation.
    C. Typical headache comes on within an hour or two of anaesthesia or coming in first three post-operative days.
    D. All of the above.

39. **The most commonly affected cranial nerve after spinal anaesthesia, producing an unusual complication is :** AIIMS 1984
    A. 10th nerve
    B. 4th nerve
    C. 6th nerve
    D. 1st nerve

40. **Following spinal Anaesthesia, paralysis of every cranial nerve has been reported with the exception of :** PGI 1985
    A. 2nd and 4th nerves
    B. 9th and 11th nerves
    C. 3rd and 8th nerves
    D. 1st and 10th nerves

41. **Treatment of post-spinal Headache Prophylactically include :** AMU 1986
    A. Use of 22-24 SW gauge Needle.
    B. Separation rather than cutting of longitudinal fibers of dura, by situation of needle bavel.
    C. Adoption of prone position for several hours daily.
    D. All of the above.
    E. None of the above.

42. **The following are true about spinal anaesthesia except:** AIIMS 1984
    A. The spinal tap is done at the level of the L3-L4 or L4-L5.
    B. 2% lignocaine is used.
    C. Hyperbaric solutions are used.
    D. Height of the analgesia is dependent upon site of injection, volume, dose and position of the patient.

43. **All the following are signs of local anaesthetic toxicity except :** PGI 1982
    A. Drowsiness
    B. Convulsions
    C. Tinnitus
    D. Hypertension

44. **All of the following are effective topically except :** AP 1997
    A. Procaine
    B. Cocaine
    C. Lidocaine
    D. Amethocaine

45. **Local anaesthetics act by inhibiting :** Kerala 1997
    A. Motor fibres only
    B. Motor & sensory fibres
    C. Only sensory fibres
    D. None

46. **Etidocaine differs from Bupivacaine in that the former :** DNB 1990
    A. Used in concentration double those of Bupivacaine.
    B. Less potent for producing sensory block.
    C. Less reliable, more rapidly eliminated.
    D. More potent for motor block.
    E. All of the above.

Ans.	30. A	31. D	32. E	33. A	34. C	35. A	36. D	37. D	38. D	39. C
	40. D	41. D	42. B	43. D	44. A	45. B	46. E			

47. Ampoules of the hydrochloride salt of the following local analgesic drugs can be autoclaved repeatedly except : **AMU 1985**
A. Lignocaine
B. Mepivacaine
C. Etidocaine
D. Bupivacaine
E. None of the above

48. The most appropriate sensory level for spinal anaesthesia prior to transurethral resection of the prostate is : **PGI 1981**
A. L1
B. L3
C. S1
D. S3
E. None of the above

49. Vasoconstrictors are employed in local analgesia because it : **AIIMS 1984**
A. Retards absorption and reduce toxicity
B. Prolongs analgesic activity
C. Produces Ischaemia
D. All of the above
E. None of the above

50. All of the following statements about d-tubocurarine are true except : **MAHE 1995**
A. It is a glycoside obtained from Chondodendron tomentosum.
B. It produces non-depolarizing neuromuscular blockade of the skeletal muscle.
C. It is not absorbed when administered orally.
D. It causes histamine release and ganglion blockade.

51. All of the following statements about cocaine are true except : **MAHE 1995**
A. It is an alkaloid obtained from Erythroxylon coca
B. It is a local anaesthetic
C. It produces active mydriasis
D. It is a vasodilator

52. Drugs once in the circulation, hydrolysed by pseudocholinesterase in the plasma and liver includes none of the following except : **PGI 1985**
A. Lignocaine
B. Etidocaine
C. Procaine
D. Bupivacaine
E. Prilocaine

53. Local anaesthesia causing vasoconstriction is :
Rajasthan 1998
A. Dibucaine
B. Procaine
C. Bupivacaine
D. Carboxycaine

54. Maximum permitted dose of Lignocaine with adrenaline is——mg/kg body weight.
JIPMER 1992
A. 2
B. 3
C. 4
D. 7

55. Heavy lignocaine used in Spinal anaesthesia has a concentration of : **AIIMS 1992**
A. 1%
B. 2%
C. 2.5%
D. 5%

56. In spinal anaesthesia Bupivacaine is used is :
Delhi 1993; AIIMS 1992
A. 0.25%
B. 1%
C. 2%
D. 4%

57. First fibres to be blocked in spinal anaesthesia is :
AIIMS 1992
A. Sympathetic preganglionic
B. Afferent motor nerves
C. Sensory fibres
D. Efferent motor nerves

58. The complication seen more often in epidural anaesthesia is : **TN 1993, 96**
A. Hypotension
B. Headache
C. Urinary retention
D. Meningitis

59. The agent used in epidural anaesthesia to relieve pain is : **AI 1993**
A. Morphine
B. Diclofenac
C. Lignocaine
D. Thiopentone

60. Drugs to be avoided in epileptic patients are following except : **DNB 1995**
A. Propofol
B. Etomidate
C. Enflurane
D. Isoflurane

61. Thiopentone : **Delhi 1987**
A. Reduces cerebral metabolic rate and oxygen consumption
B. It has anti-analgesic properties
C. Acute tolerance
D. All are true

62. Combination of local anaesthetic with adernaline :
Delhi 1987
A. Increases the depth of block
B. Increases the area of block
C. Increases the time duration of block
D. Decreases the dosage of local anaesthetic

63. Making the spinal anaesthetic solution hyperosmolar is to : **AMC 1986**
A. Make the block more quick acting
B. Increase the depth of block
C. Prolong the duration of block
D. Limit the extent of block

64. Local anaesthesia is contraindicated in :
AIIMS 1988
A. Haemophilia
B. Intermittent claudication
C. Diabetic gangrene of foot
D. All of the above

Ans.	47. E	48. E	49. D	50. A	51. D	52. C	53. B	54. D	55. D	56. A
	57. A	58. A	59. A	60. D	61. D	62. C	63. D	64. A		

65. **Non-depolarising muscle relaxants is :**
                                       Kerala 1998
   A. Scoline   B. Atracurim
   C. Vecuromium   D. Both B and C

66. **In epidural anaesthesia by opioid, site of action is:**
                                       AIIMS 1998
   A. Substantia gelatinosa   B. CNS
   C. Spinal sensory nerve   D. Ventral rami

67. **Which local anaesthetic is most cardiotoxic :**
                                     JIPMER 1997
   A. Bupivacaine   B. Procaine
   C. Lidocaine   D. Chlorprocaine

68. **Subarachnoid block as anaesthesia is contraindi-cated in :**   **AIIMS 1984, 87**
   A. Diabetic gangrene
   B. Buerger's disease
   C. Atherosclerotic gangrene
   D. Full stomach
   E. Hemophilia

69. **Lignocaine can cause :**   **UPSC 1987**
   A. Cardiac arrest   B. Syncope
   C. Convulsions   D. All of the above

70. **Spinal segments required to be blocked during epidural anaesthesia for obstetric analgesia is :**
                                       Delhi 1995
   A. T11-12 and L1-4   B. T9-10
   C. T10-12   D. L1-4

71. **Most common complication of spinal anaesthesia is :**   **UPSC 1984**
   A. Post-spinal headache   B. Arrythmias
   C. Hypotension   D. Meningitis

72. **One of the following affected by local anaesthetics first :**   **AI 1995**
   A. Type-II   B. A
   C. B   D. C

73. **Which of the following is not an advantage of epidural over spinal anaesthesia :**   **Orissa 1998**
   A. Does not cause meningitis
   B. Less spinal headache
   C. Less post-spinal hypotension
   D. Short acting

74. **Which of the following is maximum protein bound :**
                                       AMU 1986
   A. Mepivacaine   B. Bupivacaine
   C. Prilocaine   D. Lignocaine

75. **Reversal of non-depolarising muscle relaxant is done by :**   **Delhi 1998**
   A. Atropine and neostigmine
   B. Atropine and glycopyrolate
   C. Atropine and pancuronium
   D. Edophonium and neostigmine

76. **Respiratory arrest under spinal anaesthetic is mostly due to :**   **PGI 1982**
   A. Intercostal paralysis
   B. Decreased cardiac output
   C. Phrenic nerve paralysis
   D. All of the above
   E. None of the above

77. **The best position for postural drainage of segment of the lower lobe is :**   **PGI 1984**
   A. 45° head down, supine
   B. 45° head down, lying on normal side
   C. Vertical, sitting
   D. Inclined forward, sitting
   E. Horizontal, pillows under hips, supine

78. **Consider the following criteria :**   **UPSC 1977**
   Ability to
   1. Lift the head for five seconds
   2. Open the eyes widely
   3. Move the arms
   4. Protrude the tongue
   Clinical criteria for assessing recovery from neuromuscular blockade would include :
   A. 1, 2 and 3   B. 2, 3 and 4
   C. 1 and 4   D. 1, 2 and 4

79. **Effect of non-depolarizing muscle relaxants is increased by :**   **Delhi 1998**
   A. Hypocalcemia   B. Hypothermia
   C. Neostigmine   D. Hyperkalemia

80. **Total spinal anaesthesia should be recognised immediately when the following signs and symptoms occur :**   **Karnataka 1987**
   A. Nausea
   B. Difficulty in phonation
   C. Headache
   D. Hypotension

81. **Vasoconstrictor drug used in local analgesia without untoward effects is :**   **Karnataka 1987**
   A. Adrenaline   B. Phenyl ephrine
   C. Noradrenaline   D. Felypressin

Ans.	65. D	66. A	67. A	68. E	69. D	70. A	71. C	72. D	73. D	74. B
	75. A	76. D	77. E	78. B	79. A	80. D	81. A			

82. When anaesthetizing for an infected index finger one of the following is contraindicated :
    Karnataka 1989
    A. Rubber tourniquet B. 2% xylocaine
    C. 0.5% adrenaline D. Ring block

83. About Lidocaine, all is true except : Delhi 1994
    A. Dose needs to be altered in renal failure
    B. Loading dose before continuous infusion
    C. Prolongs refractory period
    D. It is very little affected by heat and pH

84. Tuohy's needle is used for : Delhi 1994
    A. Spinal analgesia B. Lumbar puncture
    C. Liver biopsy D. Lung biopsy

85. Antinociception without profound inhibition of motor activity regardless of anaesthetic technique employed is best achieved with : DNB 1990
    A. Lignocaine B. Cinchocaine
    C. Prilocaine D. Bupivacaine

86. Shortest acting local anaesthetic is :
    Rajasthan 1990
    A. Procaine B. Bupivacaine
    C. Zylocaine D. Chlorprocaine

87. Which is the most potent local anaesthetic among the following : Rajasthan 1990, 94
    A. Tetracaine B. Dibucaine
    C. Neubacaine D. Lignocaine

88. Spontaneous release of acetylcholine at NM junction produces : AI 1995
    A. Miniature action potential
    B. Junctional potential
    C. Action potential
    D. Any of the above

89. In morphine epidural anaesthesic, analgesic effect occurs in : Delhi 1995
    A. 0-2 hours B. 2-6 hours
    C. 6-12 hours D. 12-24 hours

90. Dose of morphine for epidural induction (in mg) is :
    Delhi 1995
    A. 0.1-1.0 B. 2-3
    C. 3-5 D. 5-7

91. Local anaesthesia which is antimuscarinic on heart muscle receptors is : Delhi 1995
    A. Procaine B. Cocaine
    C. Chloroprocaine D. None of the above

92. Earliest sign of systemic absorption of local anaesthetic is : TN 1996
    A. Convulsions B. Circumoral numbness
    C. Circulatory collapse D. Respiratory arrest

93. Neuromuscular blockade caused by all except :
    Kerala 1996
    A. Gentamicin B. Histamine
    C. Succinyl choline D. d-tubocuraine

94. The sequence of recovery from local anaesthesia is :
    JIPMER 1997
    A. Presymp. ganglionic, Proprioception, motor
    B. Motor, pro, Presymp. ganglionic
    C. Presymp, Motor, proprioception
    D. Proprio, Motor, Presymp. ganglionic

95. Competitive cholinergic blocker : Delhi 1996
    A. Suxamethonium B. Ganglion blocker
    C. Decamethonium D. Dantrotene

96. Ipratropium bromide produces following except :
    AI 1996
    A. Bronchoconstriction
    B. IOT
    C. Does not depress mucociliary clearance
    D. Bad taste is a side effect

97. Following is reversible NM blocking agent :
    AI 1996
    A. d-TC B. Echothiophate
    C. Metocurine D. Gallamine

98. To increase the duration of spinal anaesthesia all of the following are used except : Rajasthan 1994
    A. Tetracaine instead of lidocaine
    B. Adrenaline
    C. Phenylephrine
    D. 10% Dextrose

99. In sub-arachnoid block which recovers last :
    WB 1998
    A. Pin prick
    B. Sympathetic
    C. Visceral motor activity
    D. Proprioception

100. Effect of non-depolarizing muscle relaxants is increased by : Delhi 1998
    A. Hypocalcemia B. Hypothermia
    C. Neostigmine D. Hyperkalemia

101. All of the following are advantages of epidural anaesthesia over spinal anaesthesia except :
    Orissa 1998
    A. Dural puncture is avoided
    B. Chances of meningitis are very low
    C. Post-spinal headache is avoided
    D. Its duration of action is very short

102. Which one of the following muscle relaxant is the shortest acting : Orissa 1998
    A. Tubocurarine B. Pancuronium
    C. Suxamethonium D. Vecuronium

Ans.	82. C	83. A	84. A	85. C	86. D	87. B	88. C	89. B	90. D	91. B
	92. B	93. B	94. A	95. B	96. A	97. B	98. D	99. A	100. A	101. D
	102. C									

103. Which of the following is a muscle relaxant :
    Orissa 1999
    A. Etomidate   B. Vecuronium
    C. Propanidid   D. Acetylcholine

104. All the following are intravenous anaesthetic agents except :   **Karnataka 1999**
    A. Ketamine   B. Midazolam
    C. Pethidine   D. Propofol

105. The dose of 5% Xylocaine in Spinal Anaesthesia for a Caesarean section is :   **Karnataka 1999**
    A. 1.8 ml   B. 1.4 ml
    C. 1.2 ml   D. 0.8 ml

106. Succinylcholine should not be used in :
    Karnataka 1999
    A. Burns of long duration
    B. Extensive muscle injuries
    C. Musculoskeletal disorders
    D. All of the above

107. True about endotracheal tube in infants is :
    AIIMS 1999
    A. Curved blade with cuffed tube
    B. Straight blade with cuffed tube
    C. Curved blade with uncuffed tube
    D. Straight blade with uncuffed tube

108. Muscle relaxant can be used in renal failure :
    PGI 1999
    A. Ketamine   B. Atracuovium
    C. Pancuronium   D. Fentanyl

109. Negative pressure in extradural space is found in what percentage of population :   **Kerala 1999**
    A. 35%   B. 65%
    C. 80%   D. 100%

110. Short acting L.A. :   **PGI 2000**
    A. Procaine   B. Lignocaine
    C. Bupivacaine   D. Tetracaine

111. Myaesthenics are resistant to following muscle relaxant :   **PGI 2000**
    A. Suxamethonium   B. Pancurium
    C. Atracuronium   D. Vecuronium

112. Saddle anaesthesia involves :   **MAHE 2000**
    A. Bilateral inferior rectal nerve block.
    B. Injecting hyperbaric ligocaine in the subdural space with patient sitting.
    C. Injecting hyperbaric local anaesthetic in the epidural space with patient sitting.
    D. Injecting hyperbaric ligocaine in the subdural space with patient in left lateral position.

113. Caudal anaesthesia is :   **MAHE 2000**
    A. Injecting local anaesthetic into the sacral hiatus.
    B. Is preferred in elderly.
    C. Injecting hyperbaric ligocaine in the subdural space with patient sitting.
    D. None of the above.

114. Which one of the following is correctly matched :
    TNPSC 1996
    A. Suxamethonium   i.   Local anaesthetic
    B. Pancuronium   ii. Muscle relaxant
    C. Lignocaine   iii. Ionotrope
    D. Bupivacaine   iv   Chronotrope

115. Local anaesthesia affects maximally to :
    UP 1999
    A. A-fibres   B. B-fibres
    C. C-fibres   D. Equally in all

116. Which of the following is not seen during extradural block :   **UP 2000**
    A. Hypotension   B. Headache
    C. Bachache   D. Meningitis

117. Thiopentone in mostly used in anaesthetic :
    Rohtak 2001
    A. It cause smooth indication
    B. Does not affect circulation
    C. Does not affect respiration
    D. Does not affect pain sensation

118. Suxamethonium action produced by:
    Rohtak 2001
    A. Thiopentone   B. Propanidid
    C. OC   D. Edrophonium

119. Local anaesthetic contraindicated in IVRA (Intravenous regional anaesthesia) :   **Kerala 2001**
    A. Bupivacaine   B. Lidocaine
    C. Prilocaine   D. Mepivacaine

120. Which of the following is drug of choice in bupivacaine induced VT :   **Kerala 2001**
    A. Lidocaine   B. Phenytoin
    C. Digoxin   D. Quinidine

121. Maximum dose of xylocaine for local anaesthesia is :
    Rajasthan 2001
    A. 200 mg   B. 250 mg
    C. 300 mg   D. 500 mg

122. Maximum dose of chloroprocaine for local infiltration and blocks is :   **Delhi 2001**
    A. 50 mg   B. 150 mg
    C. 500 mg   D. 1000 mg

Ans.	103. B	104. C	105. D	106. D	107. C	108. B	109. C	110. A	111. A	112. D
	113. A	114. B	115. C	116. A	117. A	118. B	119. A	120. A	121. C	122. D

123. **Local anaesthetics cannot be used at the site of infections because it causes :**   MAHE 2001
    A. Spread of infection   B. Lowered efficiency
    C. Both   D. None

124. **All are pre-anaesthetic medications except :**
                                              CMC 2001
    A. Atropine   B. Antihistaminics
    C. Barbiturates   D. Benzodiazepines

125. **Local anaesthesia acts by :**   A.P.-2002
    A. Inhibiting Na+ influx
    B Inhibiting K+ efflux
    C. Opening K+ channels
    D. Cl- channel mediated effect

126. **The topical use of following local anaesthetic is not recommended :**   AIIMS 2002
    A. Lignocaine   B. Bupivacaine
    C. Cocaine   D. Dibucaine

127. **Interscalene approach to brachial plexus block does not provide optimal surgical anaesthesia in the area of distribution of which of the following nerve :**
                                              AI 2003
    A. Musculocutaneous   B. Ulnar
    C. Radial   D. Median

128. **In all of the following conditions neuroaxial blockade is absolutely contraindicated except :**   AI 2003
    A. Patient refusal
    B. Coagulopathy
    C. Severe hypovolemia
    D. Pre-existing neurological deficits

129. **Adrenaline is not used along with local anaesthesia in which of the following areas :**   JIPMER 2003
    A. Epidural space   B. Lower limb
    C. Penis   D. Back

130. **A patient undergoing caesarean section following prolonged labour under subarachnoid block developed carpopedal spasm. Lignocaine was used as anaesthetic agent. The most likely diagnosis is:**   AI 2004
    A. Amniotic fluid embolism
    B. Lignocaine toxicity
    C. Hypocalcemia
    D. Hypokalemia

131. **Bupivacaine :**   Karnataka 2005
    A. Causes depolarization of nerve membranes.
    B. Has a shorter duration of action thallignocaine.
    C. Is unsuitable for intrathecal use.
    D. Is contraindicated for intravenous regional anaesthesia (IVRA).

132. **Order of sensitivity of nerve fibres to Local anaesthetic in decreasing order :**   AIIMS 2008
    A. Pain (C and A-delta), Preganglionic sympathetic (B), motor
    B. Preganglionic sympathetic (B), Pain (C and A-delta), sensory, motor
    C. Pain (C and A-delta), sensory, motor, Preganglionic sympathetic (B)
    D. Preganglionic sympathetic (B) sensory, motor, Pain (C and A-delta)

133. **Paravertebral black, can extend into all except :**
                                              AI 2009
    A. Sub-arachnoids space
    B. Epidural space
    C. Superior and inferior paravertebral space
    D. Inter costal space

134. **Sodium Bicarbonate given as an adjunct to local anaesthetics because :**   AI 2009
    A. ↑ onset faction and ↑ duration
    B. ↓ onset faction and ↑ duration
    C. ↓ onset faction and ↓ duration
    D. ↑ onset faction and ↓ duration

135. **Signs of successful Stellate ganglion block all except :**   AI 2009
    A. Miosis
    B. Guttmann sign
    C. Bradycardia
    D. Unilateral nasal stuffiness

Ans. 123. B   124. C   125. A   126. B   127. B   128. D   129. C   130. B   131. D   132. B
      133. A   134. A   135. C

EXPLANATIONS OF LOCAL ANAESTHESIA

1. Ans. — D. Incontinence of urine

2. Ans. — B. Prilocaine

3. Ans. — A. Bretylium

4. Ans. — A. 1st and 10th

5. Ans. — A. Lidocaine

   It is used for extradural analgesia 15 ml of 2% or 20 ml of 1.5% solution and for intradural block, 1-2 ml of heavy 4% solution.

6. Ans. — C. Shrinks intestines so that other viscera are seen well.

7. Ans. — C. Type of drug used

8. Ans. — A. Respiratory paralysis

9. Ans. — D. Fall in blood pressure in epidural block is more when compared to spinal block.

10. Ans. — A. Patients in hypovolemia

11. Ans. — B. Anterior spinal artery syndrome

12. Ans. — B. Refrigeration Analgesia

13. Ans. — E. All of the above

14. Ans. — C. Mivacurium

    Mivacurium is a benzylisoquinolinium compound. Duration of action is approximately twice that of suxamethonium. Dose is 0.15-0.25 mg/kg and onset time 3.5 min with a duration of 10-15 min. The duration of action of Gallamine is 30-60 min, Alcuronium 20-60 min and Pancuronium is 20-30 min. Read pharmacokinetic properties of neuromuscular blocking drugs from table in K.D. Tripathi's Essentials of Medical Pharmacology.

15. Ans. — A. Fluid (spinal) is alternately withdrawn and reinjected under pressure.

16. Ans. — D. Hyperbaric

17. Ans. — D. All of the above

18. Ans. — D. A and B are true

19. Ans. — B. Normal CSF pressure

20. Ans. — C. Large quantitiy of IV fluids with foot end of bed elevated.

    Other methods which may help are lying down of the patient with foot end of bed raised, in semidarkness about 6 hours after operation. Reading and smoking prohibited for a further six-hours. The administration of codeine or pethidine is helpful and patient should be encouraged to drink as much as possible.

21. Ans. — B. Does not cross blood brain-barrier

22. Ans. — B. Subdural space

23. Ans. — D. Extradural space

24. Ans. — C. L3-L4 vertebrae

25. Ans. — D. Solutions can be autoclaved

    Adrenaline does not greatly prolong its effect but reduces its toxicity. Mixing with Dextran-150 prolongs its effects.

26. Ans. — C. Prilocaine

    Prilocaine was described by Lofgren and Tegner, tested pharmacologically by Wielding and used clinically by Gordh in 1959. Methhemoglobin is continuously formed in Red cell metabolism but normally does not exceed 1% of hemoglobin at a time. The presence of cyanosis indicates that 1.5 g/dl or more of hemoglobin is circulating as methaemoglobin.

27. Ans. — C. Bupivacaine

28. Ans. — C. No motor paralysis

29. Ans. — D. Adrenaline

30. Ans. — A. Is old

31. Ans. — D. All of the above

32. Ans. — E. All of the above

33. Ans. — A. Height of the patient

34. Ans. — C. 3-4 days

35. Ans. — A. 1st post-operative day

Post-lumbar puncture headache occurs in upto 20% of patients and upto 75% of patients with a large size (e.g. a Tuohy) needle penetrates the dura. Onset in first three post-operative days. Usually worse when the patient sits or stands. Sicard first suggested in 1902 that cause might be leakage of CSF into epidural space and average loss is about 10 ml/h and healing (according to radioisotope myelography) may take 3 weeks.

36. Ans. — D. Cauda equina syndrome

37. Ans. — D. Motor and proprioceptive in high concentration

38. Ans. — D. All of the above

39. Ans. — C. 6th nerve

40. Ans. — D. 1st and 10th nerves

41. Ans. — D. All of the above

42. Ans. — B. 2% lignocaine is used

43. Ans. — D. Hypertension

44. Ans. — A. Procaine

Procaine is used for local infiltration— 0.25-1% and for nerve block 1-2%. It was synthesized by Alfred Einhorn (1856 - 1917). It is the agent of choice in patients with a history of malignant hyperpyrexia (Procaine intravenously is used for malignant hyperpyrexia, in almost toxic doses).

45. Ans. — B. Motor & sensory fibres

46. Ans. — E. All of the above

47. Ans. — E. None of the above

48. Ans. — E. None of the above

49. Ans. — D. All of the above

50. Ans. — A. It is a glycoside obtained from Chondodendron tomentosum.

51. Ans. — D. It is a vasodilator

Cocaine is a vasoconstrictor. It is therefore used in spray to produce ischemia of nose e.g. before nasal intubation.

52. Ans. — C. Procaine

53. Ans. — B. Procaine

54. Ans. — D. 7

55. Ans. — D. 5%

56. Ans. — A. 0.25%

57. Ans. — A. Sympathetic preganglionic

Order of blocking nerve fibres are autonomic preganglionic B fibres, temperature fibres-cold before warm, pin prick fibres, fibres conveying pain greater than pinprick, touch fibres, deep pressure fibres, somatic motor fibres, fibres conveying vibratory sense and proprioceptive impulses.

58. Ans. — A. Hypotension

59. Ans. — A. Morphine

It is a respiratory depressant. Fentanyl is not used epidurally but I/V. Usually 0.5% Bupivacaine is used (1.5 - 2.5 ml).

60. Ans. — D. Isoflurane

61. Ans. — D. All are true

Distribution follows bi or tri-exponential model, first phase 2-4 min, second phase 40-50 min. Thiopentone metabolism begins after 15 min. Its elimination half life is 9h.

62. Ans. — C. Increases the time duration of block

63. Ans. — D. Limit the extent of block

64. Ans. — A. Haemophilia

65. Ans. — D. Both B and C

66. Ans. — A. Substantia gelatinosa

67. Ans. — A. Bupivacaine

Bupivacaine is more prone to induce ventricular tachycardia and cardiac depression and therefore should not be used for intravenous regional analgesia.

68. Ans. — E. Hemophilia

69. Ans. — D. All of the above

70. Ans. — A. T11-12 and L1-4

71. Ans. — C. Hypotension

Hypotension is below 80-90 mmHg systolic.

72. Ans. — D. C

The minimum concentration of local drug necessary to cause block of a nerve fibre of given diameter is known as the Cm. Sequence of block in regional analgesia is autonomic, sensory and finally motor according to fibre diameter.

73. Ans. — D. Short acting

74. Ans. — B. Bupivacaine

75. Ans. — A. Atropine and neostigmine

76. Ans. — D. All of the above

77.   Ans. — E.   Horizontal, pillows under hips, supine

78.   Ans. — B.   2, 3 and 4

79.   Ans. — A.   Hypocalcemia

80.   Ans. — D.   Hypotension

81.   Ans. — A.   Adrenaline

82.   Ans. — C.   0.5% adrenaline

83.   Ans. — A.   Dose needs to be altered in renal failure

84.   Ans. — A.   Spinal analgesia

85.   Ans. — C.   Prilocaine

86.   Ans. — D.   Chlorprocaine

87.   Ans. — B.   Dibucaine

88.   Ans. — C.   Action potential

The action is blocked by depolarizing agents, non-depolarising agents and toxins.

89.   Ans. — B.   2-6 hours

90.   Ans. — D.   5-7

91.   Ans. — B.   Cocaine

92.   Ans. — B.   Circumoral numbness

93.   Ans. — B.   Histamine

94.   Ans. — A.   Presymp. ganglionic, Proprioception, motor

95.   Ans. — B.   Ganglion blocker

96.   Ans. — A.   Bronchoconstriction

Ipratropium bromide is found to be effective in asthmatic bronchitis and COPD (by causing bronchodilation).

97.   Ans. — B.   Echothiophate

Ecothiopate is an anticholinesterase.

98.   Ans. — D.   10% Dextrose

99.   Ans. — A.   Pin prick

100.   Ans. — A.   Hypocalcemia

101.   Ans. — D.   Its duration of action is very short

102.   Ans. — C.   Suxamethonium

103.   Ans. — B.   Vecuronium

104.   Ans. — C.   Pethidine

105.   Ans. — D.   0.8 ml

For spinal analgesia, lignocaine is used in strengths of 2% plain or 5% with dextrose 3.0 and 7.5%

106.   Ans. — D.   All of the above

107.   Ans. — C.   Curved blade with uncuffed tube

108.   Ans. — B.   Atracurium

Atracurium has Hofmann degradation and alkaline ester hydrolysis in the plasma and elsewhere in the body. Elimination half-life is 20 min.

109.   Ans. — C.   80%

110.   Ans. — A.   Procaine

111.   Ans. — A.   Suxamethonium

112.   Ans. — D.   Injecting hyperbaric ligocaine in the subdural space with patient in left lateral position.

113.   Ans. — A.   Injecting local anaesthetic into the sacral hiatus.

114.   Ans. — B.   Pancuronium   ii)   Muscle relaxant

115.   Ans. — C.   C-fibres

116.   Ans. — A.   Hypotension

Hypotension (below 80-90 mm Hg) and gross hypertension are contraindications. There may be fall of CSF pressure.

117.   Ans. — A.   It cause smooth indication

118.   Ans. — B.   Propanidid

119.   Ans. — A.   Bupivacaine

120.   Ans. — A.   Lidocaine

121.   Ans. — C.   300 mg

122.   Ans. — D.   1000 mg

123.   Ans. — B.   Lowered efficiency

124.   Ans. — C.   Barbiturates

125.   Ans. — A.   Inhibiting Na+ influx

126.   Ans. — B.   Bupivacaine

127.   Ans. — B.   Ulnar

Interscalene approach to brachial plexus does not provide optimal surgical anaesthesia in the area of distribution of Ulnar nerve.

128.   Ans. — D.   Pre-existing neurological deficits

Absolute contraindications for Spinal blockade :

a)   Patient refusal to proceed is trespass.

b)   Shock - Severe hypovolumia, dehydration, Hypotension < 80-90 mm Hg systolic, Gross hypertension.

c)   Uncorrected coagulopathy or Anticoagulation - It may promote the occurrence of epidural haematoma.

d)   Raised Intracranial pressure - Dural puncture carries the risk of tentorial/medullary herniation.

129.   Ans. — **C.**   Penis

For doing surgery block of digits, penis or external ear, adrenaline is not used.

130.   Ans. — **B.**   Lignocaine toxicity

131.   Ans. — **D.**   Is contraindicated for intravenous regional anaesthesia (IVRA).

132.   Ans. — **B.**   Preganglionic sympathetic (B), Pain (C and A-delta), sensory, motor

133.   Ans. — **C.**   Superior and inferior paravertebral space

134.   Ans. — **A.**   ↑ onset faction and - duration

*   **Onset correlate with pKa**
*   **Potency correlates with lipid solubility**
*   **Duration correlates with degree of protein**
*   **Locl anaesthetics with a pKa closet to physiological Ph will have a higher concentration of nonionized base that can pass through the nerve cell membrane and generally a more rapid onset.**

135.   Ans. — **C.**   Bradycardia

Stellate ganglion block :

Indications

1. *Pain syndrome.*

CPRS type 1 and 2

Refractory angina

Phantom limb pain

2. *Vascular insufficiency*

Raynauds syndrome

Scleoderma

Frostibite

Obliterative vascular disease.

4

IMPORTANT TEXT OF GENERAL ANAESTHESIA

CLASSIFICATION OF GENERAL ANAESTHETICS

A.   Inhalation of general anaesthetics

a) Gases

— Cyclopropane
— N_2O (nitrous oxide)

b) Volatile liquids

(i) Ether (diethyl ether)
(iii) Ethylchloride
(v) Chloroform

(ii) Trichloroethylene
(iv) Enflurane
(vi) Halothane

B.   I.V. General anaesthetics

a) *Barbiturates (ultra-short acting)*

— Sodium pentothal (thiopental Na)
— Methohexital

b) *Non-Barbiturates:*

i   Steroid- Althesin
iii Etomidate

ii   Eugenol derivative- Propanidid
vi   Phencyclidine derivative- Ketamine

PROPERTIES OF ANAESTHETIC AGENTS USED

Agent	*Boiling point*	*Partition coefficient*
Cyclopropane	-33°C	—
Liquid Ether	35° C	15
Nitrous oxide	-89° C	—
Chloroform	61°C	—
Halothane	50°C	2.3
Methoxyflurane	104° C	13
Trilene	87° C	—

CONCENTRATIONS OF VARIOUS ANAESTHETIC AGENTS USED

A.   *General Anaesthetics*

Agent	*Concentration*
Ether	5-15% (10-15% for induction; 4-5% for maintenance)
Chloroform	0.5-1.0%
Halothane	1-4%
Methoxyflurane	0.75%
Fluorexene	3.4%
N_2O	3.4%
Cyclopropane	15-25% (induction); 10-15% (maintenance)
Trichlorethylone	0.5%

B.　*Local Anaesthetics*

	Surface	Infiltration	Nerve block
Procaine	—	0.5%	1%
Prilocaine	—	0.5%	1%
Lignocaine	2-4%	0.5%	1%
	(Tonometry-4%)		(Spinal-5%)

ANALGESICS FOR MAINTENANCE OF ANAESTHESIA

1.　*FENTANYL*

Indications

As a supplement to nitrous oxides anaesthesia. It does not cause hypotension and is useful for patients with cardiovascular instability.

Contraindications :
1. MAOI therapy.
2. Liver failure.
3. Obstetric anaesthesia immediately prior to delivery of the baby.
4. Head injury.

Relative contraindication :

Patients prone to post-operative respiratory depression.

Dosage :
1. Spontaneous respiration: 0.005-0.2 mg IV given over 10 minutes lasts approximately 1 hour.
2. IPPV: 0.2-0.5 mg IV at the beginning of an operation provides analgesia for 30-60 minutes. Give 0.005 mg increments when indicated. A dose of 50 g/Kg IV provides sufficient analgesia for operations lasting for 4-6 hours. **Doses should be reduced for elderly, ill or myxoedematous patients.**

Complications :
1. Respiratory depression (may occur several hours after recovery from anaesthesia).
2. Muscular rigidity.
3. Transient hypotension.
4. Bradycardia.
   The incidence of these complications is reduced by giving each dose slowly over 10 minutes.

2.　*PHENOPERIDINE*

Indications :
1. As a supplement to nitrous oxide anaesthesia for ventilated patients whose operation will last at least within 2 hours.
2. Suitable for patients with cardiovascular instability.

Contraindications :
1. MAOI therapy
2. Liver failure
3. Obstetric anaesthesia immediately prior to delivery of the baby.
4. Head injury.

Relative contraindication :

Patients prone to post-operative respiratory depression.

Dosage :

Give 2-4 mg at the beginning of anaesthesia, and 1 mg increments when indicated.

Complications :
1. Respiratory depression
2. Bradycardia
3. Hypotension (very rarely)

MUSCLE RELAXANTS FOR MAINTENANCE OF ANAESTHESIA

NB : All patients who have received muscle relaxants must be ventilated until adequate spontaneous respiration is established. Never permit a patient to be paralysed without supplementary agents to produce anaesthesia.

1. *SUXAMETHONIUM INFUSION*

Indications :

Operations lasting less than 1 hour where paralysis with only minimal relaxation of the abdominal muscles is required (e.g. gynaecological procedures, laparoscopy and bronchoscopy).

Absolute contraindications :

1. History of malignant hyperpyrexia.
2. Serum potassium greater than 5.5 mmol/L.
3. Penetrating eye injury.
4. Myasthenia gravis.
5. Myotonia.
6. Paraplegia or quadriplegia associated with active muscle wasting.
7. Massive muscle trauma.
8. Burns in the period of 1 week to 2 months after the burn.
9. Renal failure with untreated hyperkalemia.

Relative contraindications :

1. Liver disease.
2. Plasma cholinesterase deficiency.

Premedication :

Give atropine 0.6 mg IV at induction.

Dosage :

1. Intubation: 1-2 mg/kg.
2. Maintenance: 0.1% solution of suxamethonium in physiological saline at the rate of necessary to stop spontaneous efforts to breathe and movement of limbs. Usually 140-400 ml per hour is sufficient.

Complications :

1. Dual block unlikely if not more than 400 mg is given over 1 hour.
2. Tachyphylaxis.
3. Bradycardia : This follows repeated doses of suxamethonium unless atropine is given.
4. Dysrhythmias and cardiac arrest : These may be prevented by atropine premedication.
5. Increased intraocular pressure : Tubocuraine 3 mg IV given 3 minutes before the suxamethonium or acetazolamide 500 mg IV immediately before induction are said to prevent the increase but not everyone agrees.
6. Bronchospasm.
7. Increased serum potassium : This is the reason why it is contraindicated in certain cases.
8. Increased intracranial pressure. The increase is transient and its risks should be balanced against suxamethonium's other advantages.

Intermittent doses of suxamethonium

Indications

Operations lasting less than 30 minutes when paralysis is required (e.g. bronchoscopy, laparoscopy)

Contraindications

Both absolute and relative contraindications are as for suxamethonium infusion, above.

Premedication

Give atropine 0.6 mg IV at induction.

Dosage

1.   Intubation 2 mg/kg.
2.   Increments 10 mg whenever the patient shows any sign of muscle movement.

Complications

As for suxamethonium infusion, above.

2.   *ALCURONIUM*

Indications

Operations where muscle relaxation is required for at least 30 minutes.

Contraindications

1.   Previous adverse reaction to alcuronium
2.   Myasthenia gravis
3.   Myasthenic syndrome
4.   Asthma
5.   Malignant hyperpyrexia
6.   Muscle weakness
7.   Liver disease

Dosage

1.   Initially: 10-20 mg
2.   Increments: 5 mg when required

Use decreased doses for patients with renal failure or if trimethaphan is used.

Complications

1.   Respiratory paralysis
2.   Minimal hypotension
3.   Bronchospasm

3.   *PANCURONIUM*

Indications

1.   Operations where muscle relaxation is required for at least 30 minutes and an increase in blood pressure would be beneficial.
2.   Asthma
3.   Liver disease

Contraindications

1.   Myasthenia gravis
2.   Myasthenic syndrome
3.   Hypertension, whatever the cause
4.   Muscular weakness
5.   Atrial fibrillation

Dosage

1.   Initially: 0.1 mg/kg
2.   Increments 2 mg when required

Use decreased doses for patients with renal failure or if trimethaphan is used.

Complications

1.   Respiratory paralysis
2.   Hypertension
3.   Tachycardia

4.   *TUBOCURARINE*

Indications

Operations where muscle relaxation is required for at least 30 minutes and a decrease in blood pressure would be beneficial.

Contraindications

1.   Previous adverse reaction to tubocurarine.
2.   Myasthenia gravis
3.   Myasthenic syndrome
4.   Muscular weakness
5.   Asthma
6.   Malignant hyperpyrexia
7.   Liver disease.

Dosage

1.   Initially: 15-45 mg
2.   Increments: 5-10 mg when required.

    Decrease the dose for patients with renal failure or if trimethaphan is used.

Complications

1.   Respiratory paralysis
2.   Hypotension
3.   Bronchospasm
4.   Anaphylaxis- complications (2) and (3) are very severe.

Maintenance of anaesthesia

1.   Decide whether the patient is to be ventilated or allowed to breathe spontaneously.
2.   Ensure that the patient is asleep by giving inhalational agent(s) and/or an analgesic.
3.   Provide muscle relaxation if it is required by the surgeon.

DIFFERENCES BETWEEN TUBOCURARE AND SUCCINYLCHOLINE

		Tubocurare (Pachycurare)	*Succinylcholine (Leptocurare)*
1.	Effect on cathodal current	↓	↑
2.	Effect on anodal current	↑	↓
3.	Muscle contraction	Poorly sustained	Well sustained
4.	Action on motor end plate of ach	Blocks action	Produces persistent depolarization
5.	Initial excitation of skeletal muscle	Absent	Transient fasiculations
6.	Interaction with anticholinesterase	Antagonism	No antagonism
7.	Effect on prior		
	d-TC	Additive	Antagonistic
	succinylcholine	Indifference/Antagonism	Tachyphylaxis

MCQ's OF GENERAL ANAESTHESIA

> ### What is important in General Anaesthesia
>
> Agents (Ether, Halothane, N₂O, Cyclopropane, Methoxyflurane, Trilene, Chloroform, Enflurane,
> Isoflurane, Fluorexene), Properties (colours of cylinders), Benefits, Drawbacks and contraindications,
> Maintenance (analgesics e.g. Fentanyl, Muscle relaxants e.g. Scoline, d-TC, Suxamethonium,
> Alcuronium, Pancuronium, Atracurium, Vecuronium)

4-A. THEORIES & STAGES

1. The gas with the greatest solubility in blood is :
   DNB 1990
   A. Nitrogen   B. Nitrous oxide
   C. Methane   D. Hydrogen
   E. Oxygen

2. Potency of an anaesthetic agent is determined by :
   PGI 1997
   A. Blood gas coefficient   B. MAC
   C. Lipid solubility   D. Combustibility

3. Malignant hyperthermia is most commonly precipitated by :   **AIIMS 1992, 96; AI 1994**
   A. Succinyl choline   B. Dantrolene sodium
   C. Gallamine   D. Pancuronium

4. Sodalime circuit is not used in anaesthesia with :
   Delhi 1992; AIIMS 1992; AI 1993
   A. Enflurane   B. Isoflurane
   C. Trichloro ethylene D. Methoxyflurane

5. Colour of oxygen cylinder is :   **AIIMS 1992**
   A. Blue   B. Orange
   C. Black and white   D. Purple

6. The activity of muscles of eyeball during ether anaesthesia is well marked in :   **UPSC 1987**
   A. Stage-I   B. Stage-II
   C. Stage-III   D. Stage-IV

7. Induction of Anaesthesia means :   **PGI 1984**
   A. Inroduction of subject of Anaesthesia.
   B. Introduction of gases in Anaesthesia.
   C. Rendering the patient unconscious and unreactive to pain.
   D. Discussing the Anaesthesia with the patient.

8. During general anaesthesia, which of the following nerves is least likely to be affected by compression injuries :   **DNB 1991**
   A. Optic   B. Radial
   C. Median   D. Ulnar
   E. Common peroneal

9. During general anaesthesia which of the following is most common :   **Delhi 1982, 85**
   A. Sinus arrhythmia
   B. Nodal rhythm
   C. Ventricular extra-systoles
   D. Auricular extra-systoles

10. Post-anaesthetic shivering may increase metabolic rate by a factor of :   **DNB 1991**
    A. 5   B. 4
    C. 3   D. 2

11. Second stage of general anaesthesia is characterized by :   **PGI 1989**
    A. Loss of consciousness
    B. Presence of automatic movements
    C. Coherent/Incoherent shouting by the patient
    D. All of the above
    E. None of the above

12. Third stage of general anaesthesia is characterized by :   **UPSC 1992**
    A. Stage of surgical anaesthesia
    B. Stage of medullary paralysis
    C. Both the above
    D. None of the above

Ans.	1. B	2. B	3. A	4. C	5. C	6. A	7. C	8. B	9. C	10. A
	11. D	12. A								

13. Depth of anaesthesia by inhalational anesthetics depends upon :   AIIMS 1984
    A. Blood concentration of anaesthetic agent
    B. Solubility of anaesthetic agent in blood
    C. Respiratory minute volume
    D. All the above
    E. None of the above

14. Characteristic of dissociative anaesthesia includes all of the following except :   AIIMS 1983; AI 1996, 98
    A. Analgesia   B. Amnesia
    C. Catatonia   D. Hypothermia

15. Pupils in Gudel stage-II are :   Rajasthan 1998
    A. Fully dilated   B. Partially dilated
    C. Normal   D. Constricted

16. The best clinical indication of stage 3 phase 4 anaesthesia is :   UPSC 1987
    A. Complete analgesia   B. Sleep
    C. Absent eyelash reflex   D. Absent eyelid reflex

17. Which of the following is an indication for introduction of inhalational analgesia during labor :   PGI 1987
    A. Beginning of 1st stage of labor
    B. Half dilated cervix
    C. Nearly fully dilated cervix
    D. 2nd stage of labor

18. First stage general anaesthesia is characterized by :   UPSC 1986
    A. Partial analgesia   B. Loss of consciousness
    C. Loss of sense of touch   D. None of the above

19. The stage of surgical anaesthesia is best indicated by :   DNB 1990
    A. Regular respiration   B. Loss of corneal reflex
    C. Loss of eyelash reflex   D. Unconsciousness

20. The measure or index of anaesthetic potency is :   TN 1990
    A. Molecular weight
    B. Boiling point
    C. Minimum alveolar concentration
    D. None of the above

21. Hyperbaric oxygen is used for :   DNB 1989
    A. CO_2 narcosis
    B. Carbon monoxide poisoning
    C. Burns
    D. Cyanide poisoning

22. Oxygen supply through pipe line from central gas supply is at the pressure of :   Kerala 1989
    A. 30 psi   B. 50 psi
    C. 100 psi   D. 60 psi

23. Intravenous induction is preferred to inhalational induction because :   AIIMS 1989
    A. Causes less side effects
    B. Blood pressure and cardiac output are better maintained
    C. There is less danger of respiratory obstruction
    D. It is quicker

24. Inhalation of 100% oxygen results in disappearance of central cyanosis in all of the following conditions, except :   AIIMS 1986, 87
    A. Tetralogy of Fallot
    B. Diffuse interstitial fibrosis
    C. Chronic obstructive lung disease
    D. Status asthmaticus

25. The treatment of hypoxic hypoxia is :   AIIMS 1987
    A. Bronchodilators   B. Hyperbaric oxygen
    C. Pure oxygen   D. Vasodilators

26. General anaesthesia does not affect :   PGI 1987
    A. I and VI cranial nerves
    B. I and X cranial nerves
    C. III and X cranial nerves
    D. V and VI cranial nerves
    E. IV and VI cranial nerves

27. Awareness of anaesthesia is prevented by :   PGI 1990
    A. Plugging of cotton in the ear
    B. ↑ N_2O concentration
    C. ↑ depth of inhalation anaesthetics
    D. ↑ The dose of muscle relaxants
    E. Use of hypebaric O_2

28. First reflex to appear in recovery of general anaesthesia :   PGI 1984; JIPMER 1988, 90
    A. Corneal   B. Conjunctival
    C. Cough   D. Swallowing

29. Which of the following is a preventable complication during inhalational anaesthesia :   PGI 1989
    A. Aspiration   B. Laryngeal injury
    C. Hypotension   D. Vocal cord palsy

30. The stage of surgical anaesthesia is best indicated by :   Delhi 1990
    A. Regular respiration   B. Loss of corneal reflex
    C. Loss of Eyelash reflex   D. Unconsciousness

31. Intubation is indicated if respiration is :   Delhi 1988
    A. Reflex type   B. Kussmaul's type
    C. Paradoxical   D. Acidotic

32. Consciousness recovery is delayed in following anaesthesia except :   WB 1996
    A. Hyperventilation   B. CO_2 narcosis
    C. Residual curare   D. Intra-operative hypoxia

Ans.	13. D	14. D	15. A	16. C	17. C	18. A	19. A	20. C	21. B	22. D
	23. D	24. A	25. C	26. B	27. C	28. D	29. A	30. A	31. C	32. A

33. All of the following are factors which slow the speed of induction except : **Delhi 1983**
    A. Respiratory depression
    B. Laryngospasm
    C. Breath holding
    D. Presence of poor circulation to nonvital organs

34. Which of the following is especially useful in children but is not stable with sodalime : **DNB 1993**
    A. Enflurane   B. Isoflurane
    C. Sevoflurane   D. Desflurane

35. Sigard Anderson normogram determines blood : **AIIMS 1983**
    A. Chloride   B. Calcium
    C. Bicarbonate   D. pO2

36. Dose of I/M Ketamine is : **AIIMS 1986**
    A. 1-2 mg/kg   B. 2-3 mg/kg
    C. 4-5 mg/kg   D. 8-10 mg/kg

37. Colour of Helium cylinder is : **PGI 1985**
    A. Blue   B. Black
    C. Orange   D. Brown

38. The concentration of CO_2 used for anaesthesia is : **Delhi 1986**
    A. 0.05%   B. 0.5%
    C. 5.0%   D. 50

39. Awakening is most rapid with : **NIMHANS 1986**
    A. Thiopentone   B. Propanidid
    C. Disoprofol   D. Etomidate

40. Laryngeal reflex is lost in ——— stage of anaesthesia. **AIIMS 1985**
    A. IIIa   B. IIIb
    C. IIIc   D. IIId

41. Inhalation of 4% ether is likely to correspond with a blood level of about : **Delhi 1984**
    A. 27 mg%   B. 36 mg%
    C. 46 mg%   D. 57 mg%

42. Stage 3, plane 4 anaesthesia is best indicated clinically by : **Delhi 1986**
    A. Dilated pupils
    B. Fixed pupils
    C. Absent thoracic respiration
    D. Absent laryngeal reflex
    E. Absent corneal reflex

43. After a patient has breathed a 75: 25 N_2O ; O_2 mixture for an hour, uptake on N_2O by the body will then be about : **AIIMS 1980**
    A. 0   B. 10 ml/min
    C. 45 ml/min   D. 85 ml/min
    E. 175 ml/min

44. In the second stage of anaesthesia the pupil is : **AIIMS 1987**
    A. Constricted   B. Partially dilated
    C. Normal in size   D. Totally dilated

45. Drugs which does not cross blood brain barrier : **AIIMS 1983**
    A. Neostigmine   B. Physostigmine
    C. Atropine   D. Hyoscaine

46. Adrenaline is contraindicated during —— anaesthesia . **AIIMS 1980, 89, 92**
    A. Thiopentone   B. Ether
    C. Trilene   D. Halothane

47. Pupillary dilatation occurs in stage 3, plane 2 with except : **UPSC 1985**
    A. Halothane   B. Ether
    C. Cyclopropane   D. Fluroxene

48. Principle causes of inadequate ventillations during anaesthesia include : **AIIMS 1989**
    A. Obstruction to air passage.
    B. Alternation is gas exchange due to the anaesthetic agent.
    C. Neuromuscular depression of respiratory mechanisms.
    D. All of the above.
    E. None of the above.

49. Following are factors likely to delay induction of inhalation anaesthenia except : **Bihar 1998**
    A. Old age   B. Heavy premedication
    C. Laryngospasm   D. None

50. Technical problems in intubation of children should be anticipated : **AIIMS 1980**
    A. Gargoylism
    B. Cystic hygroma of neck
    C. Still's disease
    D. Treacher Collins syndrome
    E. All of the above

51. Diffusion hypoxia is seen during : **AIIMS 1998**
    A. Induction of anaesthesia
    B. Recovery of anaesthesia
    C. Perioperatively
    D. Post-operatively

52. Induction with intravenous agents is faster in a patient with : **DNB 1992**
    A. ASD   B. VSD
    C. TOF   D. PDA

53. Pressure in oxygen cylinder is —— lbs. **PGI 1993**
    A. 100-500   B. 500-1000
    C. 1000-2000   D. 2000-5000

Ans.	33. D	34. C	35. C	36. C	37. D	38. C	39. B	40. C	41. A	42. C
	43. E	44. B	45. A	46. D	47. A	48. D	49. A	50. E	51. B	52. C
	53. B									

54. The potency of an inhalational anaesthetic depends on :
                                                        PGI 1999

A. Blood gas partition co-efficient
B. Oil-gas partition co-efficient
C. MAC
D. Pressure

55. Not true about blood gas partition coefficient is :
                                                        Delhi 2001

A. Sevoflurane < Isoflurane
B. Isoflurane < Englurane
C. Desflurane < Nitrous oxide
D. Sevoflurane < Desflurane

56. Statement true about soluble volatile anaesthetics is :
                                                        Delhi 2001

A. Water soluble
B. Rapid emergence
C. Reach rapid equilibrium during uptake
D. High blood gas partition coefficient

57. Upper respiratory tract infection is a common problem in children. All the following anaesthetic complications can occur in children with respiratory infections except :   **AI 2002**

A. Bacteremia
B. Halothane granuloma
C. Increased mucosal bleeding
D. Laryngospasm

| Ans. | 54. C | 55. D | 56. D | 57. B |

EXPLANATIONS OF GENERAL ANAESTHESIA

4-A. THEORIES & STAGES

1.   Ans. — B. **Nitrous oxide**

2.   Ans. — B. **MAC**

3.   Ans. — A. **Succinyl choline**

        A specific condition in which heat production exceeds heat loss in the body to cause a rise of temperature of at least 2°C/h. Among anaesthetics halothane can also cause. Bromocriptine and dantrolene are useful in treatment.

4.   Ans. — C. **Trichloro ethylene**

        It forms highly toxic product dichloro-ethylene resulting in paralysis of cranial nerves (especially 5th and 7th) and death and so never use it in closed circuit.

5.   Ans. — C. **Black and white**

6.   Ans. — A. **Stage-I**

7.   Ans. — C. **Rendering the patient unconscious and unreactive to pain.**

8.   Ans. — B. **Radial**

9.   Ans. — C. **Ventricular extra-systoles**

10. Ans. — A. **5**

11. Ans. — D. **All of the above**

12. Ans. — A. **Stage of surgical anaesthesia**

13. Ans. — D. **All of the above**

14. Ans. — D. **Hypothermia**

        It is typically produced by ketamine.

15. Ans. — A. **Fully dilated**

16. Ans. — C. **Absent eyelash reflex**

17. Ans. — C. **Nearly fully dilated cervix**

18. Ans. — A. **Partial analgesia**

19. Ans. — A. **Regular respiration**

20. Ans. — C. **Minimum alveolar concentration**

21. Ans. — B. **Carbon monoxide poisoning**

22. Ans. — D. **60 psi**

23. Ans. — D. **It is quicker**

24. Ans. — A. **Tetralogy of Fallot**

25. Ans. — C. **Pure oxygen**

26. Ans. — B. **I and X cranial nerves**

27. Ans. — C. **- depth of inhalation anaesthetics**

28. Ans. — D. **Swallowing**

29. Ans. — A. **Aspiration**

30. Ans. — A. **Regular respiration**

31. Ans. — C. **Paradoxical**

32. Ans. — A. **Hyperventilation**

33. Ans. — D. **Presence of poor circulation to nonvital organs.**

34. Ans. — C. **Sevoflurane**

35. Ans. — C. **Bicarbonate**

36. Ans. — C. **4-5 mg/kg**

37. Ans. — D. **Brown**

38. Ans. — C. **5.0%**

39. Ans. — B. **Propanidid**

40. Ans. — C. **IIIc**

41. Ans. — A. **27 mg%**

42. Ans. — C. **Absent thoracic respiration**

43. Ans. — E. **175 ml/min**

44. Ans. — B. **Partially dilated**

45. Ans. — A. **Neostigmine**

46.   Ans. — D.   Halothane

47.   Ans. — A.   Halothane

48.   Ans. — D.   All of the above

49.   Ans. — A.   Old age

50.   Ans. — E.   All of the above

51.   Ans. — B.   Recovery of anaesthesia

52.   Ans. — C.   TOF

53.   Ans. — B.   500-1000

54.   Ans. — C.   MAC

55.   Ans. — D.   Sevoflurane < Desflurane

56.   Ans. — D.   High blood gas partition coefficient

57.   Ans. — B.   Halothane granuloma

Halothane is respiratory depressant but not a bronchial irritant. The secretions are not stimulated.

4-B. MCQ's OF INDUCTION AGENTS

1. **Fastest reversible anaesthesia is when given by ——— route .**   **Delhi 1992, 99**
   A. Inhalational
   B. I/V
   C. Local anaesthesia
   D. None

2. **Ketamine has the following properties except :**
   PGI 1984; 89, 94, 2002
   A. Marked analgesic properties
   B. Increase in heart rate, cardiac output and blood pressure
   C. May cause unpleasant dreams
   D. Depresses laryngeal and pharyngeal reflexes

3. **All are true for thiopentone except :**   **PGI 1983, 90**
   A. Has no effect on myocardial contractility
   B. Has an alkaline pH of 10
   C. Causes vasodilation
   D. Causes dose dependent depression of central nervous system

4. **Ketamine is contraindicated in :**
   AMC 1990; AMC 1996; AI 1998
   A. Hypertension
   B. Eclampsia
   C. Raised intraocular tension and intracranial tension
   D. All of the above

5. **All of the following are features of diazepam, except :**
   AMU 1987
   A. Has prolonged duration of action, especially after multiple doses.
   B. No changes in cardio-pulmonary functions.
   C. The onset of action is faster than thiopentone.
   D. Venous irritation is common.

6. **Following features are true for propanidid except :**
   Rohtak 1987, 92
   A. Rapid induction and recovery
   B. Very soluble
   C. Rapidly metabolised by plasma cholinesterase
   D. Extraneous muscle movements are common

7. **The following statements are true of muscle relaxants except :**   **AMU 1984**
   A. Gallamine is contraindicated in renal failure.

   B. d-tubocurarine is safe in renal failure.
   C. Pancuronium and vecuronium have a prolonged effect in patients with hepatic cirrhosis.
   D. Succinylcholine depends on biliary renal excretion.

8. **The following statements are true except :**
   PGI 1983
   A. Succinylcholine is a depolarising muscle relaxant.
   B. Its action is brief due to its rapid hydrolysis by pseudocholinesterase.
   C. Can be safely given to patients with burns, trauma, hemiplegia and paraplegia.
   D. Its action is prolonged in individuals with genetic variant of pseudocholinesterase.

9. **Phase-II blocker is :**   **AMU 1990; AIIMS 1998**
   A. d-TC
   B. Scoline
   C. Cocaine
   D. Vecuronium

10. **The rate of biotransformation of thiopental in humans is approximately :**   **AIIMS 1983**
    A. 20% per hour
    B. 30% per hour
    C. 40% per hour
    D. 50% per hour
    E. 67% per hour

11. **In which of the following is Thiopentone contra-indicated :**   **JIPMER 1993**
    A. Diabetes mellitus
    B. Head injury
    C. Porphyria
    D. Retinal surgery

12. **The most suitable site for giving intravenous thiopentone is :**   **UPSC 1985**
    A. External jugular vein
    B. Anterior to elbow joint
    C. Anterior to wrist joint
    D. Forearm, outer aspect
    E. Back of the hand

13. **All are seen in ketamine anaesthesia except :**
    Kerala 1994
    A. Hypertension
    B. Hallucinations
    C. Bronchospasm
    D. Analgesia

14. **Pentothal sodium should be injected preferably into :**   **AIIMS 1986**
    A. Veins in antecubital fossa
    B. Neck veins
    C. Veins over outer aspect of forearm
    D. Femoral vein

Ans.	1. A	2. D	3. A	4. D	5. C	6. C	7. D	8. C	9. B	10. A
	11. C	12. D	13. C	14. C						

15. Physical properties of thiopentone include :
    AIIMS 1984
    A. Pale yellow colour   B. Smells like sulphur
    C. Bitter taste   D. Hygroscopic
    E. All of the above

16. Which of the following is produced nicely by administering safe dosage of thiopental sodium :
    AIIMS 1982
    A. Analgesia   B. Relaxation
    C. Hypnosis   D. All of the above

17. Thiopentone is an ultra short acting barbiturate because of its :   Delhi 1984
    A. Rapid breakdown
    B. Rapid metabolism
    C. Rapid elimination from blood
    D. All of the above

18. 250 mg of thiopentone was given just prior to the delivery. Thiopentone was present in :   AMU 1986
    A. Its concentration was equal in maternal and fetal blood in 2-3 minutes.
    B. Concentration fell in both mother and fetal blood synchronously.
    C. Fetus within 45 seconds.
    D. All of the above.

19. Pentothal is used in the concentration of :
    Delhi 1988
    A. 1.5%   B. 2.5%
    C. 5%   D. 10%
    E. 25%

20. Thiopentone if injected accidentally into an artery, the first symptom is :
    AIIMS 1985, 86; UPSC 1985; Delhi 1986
    A. Analgesia   B. Pain
    C. Paralysis   D. Skin ulceration

21. Enflurane causes ——— in tidal volume in spontaneously breathing patients.   DNB 1989
    A. Increase   B. Decrease
    C. No change   D. Variable response

22. Suxamethonium produces following except :
    WB 1996
    A. Hyperthermia   B. Reduced ocular pressure
    C. Bradycardia   D. Tachyphylaxis

23. Pancuronium dose for intubation is :   Delhi 1988
    A. 0.01 mg/kg   B. 0.1 mg/kg
    C. 1 mg/kg   D. 2 mg/kg

24. BP is increased by all except :   AMU 1987
    A. Suxamethonium   B. Gallamine
    C. Pancuronium   D. Alcuronium

25. Enflurane is contraindicated with :   DNB 1990
    A. Beta blockers
    B. ACE inhibitors
    C. Calcium channel blockers
    D. All of the above

26. Increased output of ADH occurs with all of the following, except :   AIIMS 1984
    A. Nitrous oxide   B. Halothane
    C. Methyoxy flurane   D. Epidural anaesthesia
    E. Thiopentone sodium

27. Advantages of thiopentone anaesthesia include all, except :   AIIMS 1981; Delhi 1985, 86
    A. Absence of stage of delirium
    B. Rapid recovery
    C. Ability to increase depth rapidly
    D. Good abdominal relaxation with safe dosage

28. Treatment of inadvertent injection of pentothal intra-arterially :   AI 1988
    A. Injection of procaine into the artery
    B. Papaverine intra-arterially
    C. Heparin- IV
    D. Stellate ganglion block
    E. All of the above

29. Following accidental intra-arterial injection of thiopentone which should not be done :   AIIMS 1980
    A. Remove the needle
    B. Intra-arterial heparin
    C. Intra-arterial papaverine
    D. Do a stellate ganglion block

30. Which is an isomer of Enflurane :
    A. Isoflurane   B. Methoxyflurane
    C. Cyclopropane   D. Halothane

Match the following (Ques 31 to 36)
    AIIMS 1984; Delhi 1994
31. Tubocurarine   A. 2-4 minutes
32. Gallamine   B. About 15 minutes
33. Pancuronium   C. About 30-50 minutes
34. Fazadinium   D. About 30 minutes
35. Suxemthonium   E. Between 20-35 minutes
36. Decamethonium   F. 25-40 minutes

37. Intravenous injection is painful in :   Delhi 2000
    A. Thiopentone   B. Ketamine
    C. Propofol   D. Althesin

Ans.   15. E   16. C   17. C   18. D   19. B   20. B   21. B   22. B   23. B   24. D
        25. A   26. D   27. D   28. E   29. A   30. A   31. C   32. E   33. F   34. D
        35. A   36. B   37. C

38. The following statements about Bupivacaine are true except :   **Kerala 2000**
    A. Must never be injected into a vein
    B. More cardiotoxic than Lignocaine
    C. 0.25 percent is effective for sensory block
    D. Long acting drug
    E. It produces methaemoglobinaemia

39. Anaesthetic agent of choice in renal failure :   **AI 2001**
    A. Methoxyflurane   B. Isoflurane
    C. Enflurane   D. None of the above

40. Which of the following is degraded by sodalime :
                                           JIPMER 2002
    A. Isoflurane   B. Enflurane
    C. Sevoflurane   D. Desflurane

41. During surgery for aortic arch aneurysm under deep hypothermic circulatory arrest, which of the following anaesthetic agent administered prior to circulatory arrest that also provides cerebral protection :
                                           AIIMS 2002
    A. Etomidate   B. Thiopental sodium
    C. Propofol   D. Ketamine

42. A 38 years old man is posted for extraction of last molar tooth under general anaesthesia as a day care case. He wishes to resume his work after 6 hrs. Which one of the following induction agents is preferred :
                                           AI 2003
    A. Thiopentone sodium   B. Ketamine
    C. Diazepam   D. Propofol

43. Induction agent that may cause adrenal cortex suppression is :   **AI 2003**
    A. Ketamine   B. Etomidate
    C. Propofol   D. Thiopentone

Ans.   38. E   39. C   40. C   41. B   42. D   43. B

EXPLANATIONS OF INDUCTION AGENTS

1. Ans. — A. Inhalational

2. Ans. — D. Depresses laryngeal and pharyngeal reflexes.

3. Ans. — A. Has no effect on myocardial contractility

4. Ans. — D. All of the above

5. Ans. — C. The onset of action is faster than thiopentone.

6. Ans. — C. Rapidly metabolised by plasma cholinesterase.

7. Ans. — D. Succinylcholine depends on biliary renal excretion.

8. Ans. — C. Can be safely given to patients with burns, trauma, hemiplegia and paraplegia.

9. Ans. — B. Scoline

10. Ans. — A. 20% per hour

11. Ans. — C. Porphyria

12. Ans. — D. Forearm, outer aspect

13. Ans. — C. Bronchospasm

    Ketamine is rapidly absorbed after oral, intramuscular or intravenous administration. The injection of therapeutic dose of ketamine produces a state of *"Dissociative anaesthesia".*

14. Ans. — C. Veins over outer aspect of forearm

    When injected accidently into artery, it causes severe pain at local site. Syringe is immediately removed (not be needle). Inject 5 ml of 1% procaine or other anaesthetic. A sympathetic block may be required to control profound spasm. Mild Perivenous injection is treated by application of heat for 24 hours and injection of 3-5 ml of 1% procaine with hyaluronidase.

15. Ans. — E. All of the above

16. Ans. — C. Hypnosis

17. Ans. — C. Rapid elimination from blood

    Distribution follows bi or tri-exponential model, first phase 2-4 min; second phase 40-50 min. Thiopentone metabolism begins after 15 min. Its elimination half life is 9h.

18. Ans. — D. All of the above

19. Ans. — B. 2.5%

20. Ans. — B. Pain

21. Ans. — B. Decrease

22. Ans. — B. Reduced ocular pressure

23. Ans. — B. 0.1 mg/kg

24. Ans. — D. Alcuronium

25. Ans. — A. Beta blockers

26. Ans. — D. Epidural anaesthesia

27. Ans. — D. Good abdominal relaxation with safe dosage.

    It is a weak muscle relaxant and causes laryngeal spasm.

28. Ans. — E. All of the above

29. Ans. — A. Remove the needle

30. Ans. — A. Isoflurane

31. Ans. — C. About 30-50 minutes

32. Ans. — E. Between 20-35 minutes

33. Ans. — F. 25-40 minutes

34. Ans. — D. About 30 minutes

35. Ans. — A. 2-4 minutes

36. Ans. — B. About 15 minutes

37. Ans. — C. Propofol

38. Ans. — E. It produces methaemoglobinaemia

39. Ans. — C. Enflurane

40. Ans. — C. Sevoflurane

41. Ans. — B. Thiopental sodium

42. Ans. — D. Propofol

*   Induction agents preferred in day-care anaesthesia are :

Propofol (MC used)

Atracurium

Vancuronium

43. Ans. — B. Etomidate

Etomidate causes the adrenal cortex suppression.

4-C. MCQ's OF AGENTS & MUSCLE RELAXANTS

1. All are non-depolarizing relaxants except :
DNB 1989, 95
A. d-tubocurarine   B. Pancuronium
C. Gallamine   D. Succinylcholine

2. Which of the following is not a circulatory effect of halothane : **BHU 1985**
A. Decrease in cardiac output.
B. Increased cerebral blood flow.
C. Decreased in myocardial oxygen consumption.
D. Increased heart rate secondary to a decrease in total peripheral resistance.
E. Increased myocardial automatically.

3. During Ether anaesthesia, severe metabolic acidosis tends to develop in : **AMU 1987**
A. Small children, possessing increased sympathetic nervous activity
B. Cushing disease
C. Cirrhosis of liver
D. All of the above
E. None of the above

4. When halothane is administered with 70% N_2O and O_2 the MAC value of halothane will be reduced by about : **AIIMS 1984**
A. 60%   B. 40%
C. 30%   D. 15%
E. 10%

5. Characteristic features of the depolarization block are except : **AIIMS 1981**
A. Fasciculation
B. The possibility of a dual block
C. Its potentiation by neostigmine
D. The presence of post-tetanic facilitation

6. All of the following are used as inhalation anaesthetic except : **Bihar 1990**
A. Nitrous oxide   B. Chloroform
C. Ether   D. Ketamine

7. The following are the adverse effects of chloroform as an anaesthetic except : **AIIMS 1984**
A. Cardiac arrest   B. Ventricular fibrillation
C. Hepatitis   D. Diffusion hypoxia

8. Which of the following is not flammable : **Delhi 1984**
A. Cyclopropane   B. Ethylene oxide
C. Ether   D. All of the above

9. Which of the following Anaesthestic agent is contraindicated in renal failure : **JIPMER 1992, 98**
A. d-Tubocurarine   B. Scoline
C. Halothane   D. Gallamine

10. The muscle relaxant acting directly on muscle is : **JIPMER 1992, 96**
A. Diazepam   B. Dantrolene
C. Decamethonium   D. d-Tubocurarine

11. Best uterine relaxation is seen with : **AIIMS 1992; PGI 1994; WB 1996**
A. Ether   B. Halothane
C. Chloroform   D. Nitrous oxide

12. Anaesthetic agent used safely in Bronchial asthma is : **PGI 1993**
A. Ether   B. Halothane
C. Enflurane   D. Chloroform

13. Most common cause of death from chloroform anaesthesia is : **JIPMER 1993**
A. Respiratory depression   B. Malignant hypertension
C. Ventricular fibrillation   D. ARDS

14. In mysthenia gravis, patient is most sensitive to : **TN 1993**
A. Neostigmine   B. Decamethonium
C. Gallamine   D. Scoline

15. Which does not sensitizes myocardium to catecholamine: **AI 1993; PGI 1996**
A. N_2O B. Halothane
C. Diethyl Ether   D. Methoxyflurane

Ans.	1. D	2. D	3. D	4. A	5. D	6. D	7. D	8. B	9. D	10. B
	11. B	12. B	13. B	14. C	15. C					

16. Increased intraocular tension is seen with :   AI 1993
   A. Trilene   B. Ketamine
   C. Halothane   D. Ether

17. Which of the following does not have analgesic action: Delhi 1993
   A. N₂O   B. Ether
   C. Halothane   D. Ketamine

18. An anaesthetic agent with boiling temperature more than water is :   Delhi 1993
   A. Halothane   B. Cyclopropane
   C. Methoxyflurane   D. TCE

19. A muscle relaxant undergoing non-enzymatic metabolism is :   Delhi 1993
   A. Alcuronium   B. Gallamine
   C. Pancuronium   D. Atracuronium

20. Shivering is seen in anaesthesia with :   Delhi 1993
   A. Halothane   B. N₂O
   C. Chloroform   D. Cyclopropane

21. Most patent I/V analgesic anaesthetic is :   Delhi 1993
   A. Ketamine   B. Etomidate
   C. Althesin   D. Pancuronium

22. Fasciculations with succinylcholine are first seen over: Delhi 1986, 93
   A. Eyelids   B. Limbs
   C. Neck   D. Abdomen

23. Following anaesthetic agent causes minimum cerebral vessel dilatation :   Delhi 1993
   A. Halothane   B. Cyclopropane
   C. Ether   D. N₂O

24. Which of the following is not metabolized but totally excreted by kidney: Delhi 1993
   A. Gallamine   B. Scoline
   C. d-Tubocurarine   D. Pancuronium

25. Dose of scoline beyond which dual block occurs is :   Delhi 1992
   A. 250 mg   B. 500 mg
   C. 750 mg   D. 1000 mg

26. Tachypnea is seen with which anaesthesia :   Delhi 1992
   A. Trilene   B. Halothane
   C. Ether   D. Propofol

27. Following administration of d-tubocurarine, the fourth which in a "train-of-four" stimulation disappears. What percent of reduction of twitch tension does this represent: ,   AIIMS 1982
   A. 50%   B. 70%
   C. 75%   D. 80%
   E. 90%

28. Muscle relaxant action of scoline is not prolonged by :   Kerala 1994
   A. Chloroform   B. Ethylchloride
   C. Enflurane   D. Halothane

29. Tubocurarine should not be used in patients receiving: Delhi 1984; TN 1989
   A. Morphine   B. Atropine
   C. Levodopa   D. Kanamycin

30. Cyclopropane tends to gravitate towards the floor because it is :   AIIMS 1986
   A. Lighter than air
   B. Heavier than air
   C. Vapour density is same as that of air
   D. None of the above

31. The required dose of a non-depolarizing muscle relaxant may be increased in :   PGI 1983
   A. Muscular dystrophy
   B. Dystrophia myotonica
   C. Burns
   D. Myasthenia gravis
   E. Familial periodic paralysis

32. Nitrous oxide is contraindicated in patients with pneumothorax, pneumopericardium or intestinal obstruction, because it :   AIIMS 1982
   A. Depresses an already compromised myocardium.
   B. Permits the use of a limited FIO2 only.
   C. Is less soluble than nitrogen.
   D. Causes the expansion of air filled body cavities.
   E. Depresses spontaneous respirations.

33. Nitrous oxide is avoided in surgery for retinal detachment with intravitreal injection of :   AIIMS 1986
   A. Saline   B. Sf6
   C. Xenon   D. Argon

34. Most soluble anaesthetic agent with highest blood gas coefficient is :   DNB 1991
   A. Methyoxyflurane B. Diethylether
   C. Isoflurane   D. Cyclopropane

35. Drugs employed in anaesthesia causing hypertension resulting in increased blood loss during surgery is/are: AIIMS 1981
   A. Ether   B. Halothane
   C. Cyclopropane   D. Trilene

36. One of the following inhalational agents causes coronary steal :   PGI 1985
   A. Halothane   B. Enfluranc
   C. Isoflurane   D. Ether

Ans.	16. B	17. C	18. C	19. D	20. A	21. A	22. A	23. D	24. A	25. B
	26. A	27. C	28. B	29. D	30. B	31. C	32. D	33. B	34. A	35. D
	36. C									

37. Lung clearance is slowest in the case of :
    DNB 1989
    A. Chloroform   B. Cyclopropane
    C. Trichlorethylene   D. Diethylether
    E. Both A and B are true

38. The effects of cyclopropane include all except :
    AIIMS 1982
    A. Respiratory depression
    B. Ventricular arrhythmia
    C. Diminution of renal blood flow
    D. Femoral vein

39. Following is the use of d-tubocurarine as a muscle relaxant :   PGI 1996
    A. Neostigmine may reverse the neuromuscular blockade.
    B. Neostigmine may potentiate neuromuscular block.
    C. The drug is not distributed to any tissue other than brain.
    D. The respiratory minute volume is slightly increased.

40. Induction of anaesthesia is fastest with which of the following :   AIIMS 1985
    A. Chloroform
    B. Halothane
    C. Cyclopropane
    D. Same with all of the above

41. The anaesthetic to be avoided in a patient requiring repeated surgery is :   AIIMS 1983
    A. Trichloroethylene   B. Diethylether
    C. Methoxyflurane   D. Halothane
    E. Nitrous oxide

42. The anaesthetic/s agent readily soluble in rubber tubing of anaesthetic machine is/are :   AIIMS 1985
    A. Ether   B. Halothane
    C. Methoxyflurane   D. Both B and C are true

43. Regarding halothane action on skeletal muscles is :
    AMU 1986
    A. Antagonising the effects of drugs which act by depolarization.
    B. Has minimal neuromuscular blocking action.
    C. Potentiates the action of non-depolarizing agents.
    D. All of the above.

44. Which of the following gas in stored under pressure in liquid form :   AIIMS 1984
    A. Cyclopropane   B. Nitrous oxide
    C. Carbon dioxide   D. All of the above

45. Anaesthesia causing shock during withdrawl is :
    Delhi 1996
    A. N₂O   B. Cyclopropane
    C. Halothane   D. Ether

46. Complications associated with the use of succinylcholine include/s :   AP 1989
    A. Myoglobinuria with renal failure
    B. Increased serum K+
    C. Malignant hyperthermia
    D. All of the above

47. The last muscle to be paralysed after d-tubocurarine administration is :   DNB 1991
    A. Intercostals   B. Eyelid
    C. Neck   D. Diaphragm

48. Suxamethonium should not be used in burn cases when the burn is :   DNB 1989
    A. 3 months to 3 years old
    B. 1 day to 10 days old
    C. 3 weeks to 3 months old
    D. 3 days to 3 weeks old

49. Which of the following is lighter than air :
    AIIMS 1982
    A. Nitrous oxide   B. Carbon oxide
    C. Oxygen   D. None of the above

50. All the following except one produce fasciculations when given parenterally :   DNB 1989
    A. Succinylcholine   B. Prostigmine
    C. Gallamine   D. Decamethonium

51. Peripheral vascular resistance is reduced with :
    AIIMS 1987
    A. Halothane   B. Cyclopropane
    C. Diethyl ether   D. All of the above

52. The dose of d-tubocurare is to be decreased with all except :   DNB 1991
    A. Halothane   B. Ether
    C. Streptomycin   D. Ephedrine

53. In children, for intubation used is :   AIIMS 1985
    A. Halothane   B. Curare
    C. Muscle relaxant   D. None of the above

54. Action of d-tubocurare is :   AIIMS 1985
    A. Competitive block of nicotinic receptor
    B. Competitive block of mucarinic receptor
    C. Depolarization of nicotinic receptors
    D. Depolarization of muscarinic receptors

55. Maximum bleeding in caesarean section will be seen if following drug is used :   AI 1989
    A. Halothane   B. Nitrous oxide
    C. Ketamine   D. Scoline

56. Antidote of d-tubocurare is :   AI 1990
    A. Atropine   B. Neostigmine
    C. Corticosteroids   D. Propranolol

Ans.	37 D	38. D	39. A	40. B	41. D	42. D	43. D	44. D	45. B	46. D
	47. D	48. A	49. A	50. C	51. A	52. D	53. C	54. A	55. A	56. B

57. **Neuromuscular blocking agent that causes fall in blood pressure is :**   **Rajasthan 1994**
    A. d-tubocurarine   B. Gallamine
    C. Pancuronium   D. Atracuronium

58. **Which of the following is false :**   **AIIMS 1984**
    A. Nitrous oxide cylinder is coloured blue.
    B. Nitrous oxide is in gaseous form in the cylinder.
    C. Pressure of nitrous oxide cylinder is 750 lbs.
    D. Oxygen cylinder has 1,950 lbs pressure.

59. **Following are contraindicated in the presence of cautery except :**   **DNB 1991**
    A. Halothane   B. Cyclopropane
    C. Ether   D. Ethylene

60. **Anaesthesia contraindicated in diabetes mellitus is :**   **Delhi 1990; DNB 1991**
    A. Ether   B. Halothane
    C. Trilene   D. Cyclopropane

61. **Diffusion Hypoxia is seen with :**   **AIIMS 1986**
    A. N_2O B. Trilene
    C. Halothane   D. Ether

62. **Catecholamines induced arrythmia are caused by :**   **DNB 1990**
    A. Trilene   B. Halothane
    C. Chloroform   D. All of the above

63. **Complications associated with the use of succinylcholine includes :**   **AIIMS 1986**
    A. Increase in serum K+
    B. Malignant hyperthermia
    C. Myoglobinuria with renal failure
    D. All of the above
    E. Only A and B are true

64. **Use of atropine prior to Neostigmine for reversal for relaxants effect includes, to prevent :**   **DNB 1990**
    A. Bradycardia   B. Gut contraction
    C. Hypotension   D. All of the above

65. **Neostigmine routinely in clinical use is :**   **AIIMS 1987**
    A. Neostigmine homa bromide
    B. Neostigmine methyl sulphate
    C. Neostigmine phosphate
    D. Neostigmine chloride
    E. Neostigmine nitrate

66. **N_2O remains as gas in the cylinder is the external temperature is less than :**   **Rajasthan 1998**
    A. -7°C   B. 15°C
    C. 0°C   D. 25°C

67. **Prevention of muscle pains after suxamethonium is by all of the following except :**   **AIIMS 1984**
    A. Pre-curarization, 3 mts before suxamethonium.

B. Tacrine
C. Use of large doses of suxamethorium
D. Vitamin C 500 mg b.d on the day of operation.
E. I.V. Lignocaine 2-6 mg/kg following thiopentone and 3 minutes before relaxant.

68. **Concerning Neostigmine resistant curarization :**   **AP 1987**
    A. Metabolic acidosis, a major factor.
    B. Accompanied by hypoventilation and tracheal tug.
    C. Failure of CVS and cerebral depression.
    D. Treat by infusion of sodium bicarbonate solution.
    E. All of the above.

69. **Increased sensitivity to non-depolarizing relaxants is seen in all of the following diseases except :**   **DNB 1990**
    A. Systemic Lupus Erythematosus
    B. Polymyostitis
    C. Bronchial Asthma
    D. Myasthenia gravis
    E. Dermatomyositis

70. **Concerning trichloroethylene all the facts are true except :**   **AIIMS 1983**
    A. It is non inflammable
    B. Provide Good Muscular Relaxation
    C. Dysrhythmias are commonly encountered
    D. Widely used in obstetrics analgesia
    E. Prolonged Recovery

71. **The pressure of ethyl chloride in its glass container is ——— mm Hg above atmospheric pressure :**   **AIIMS 1985**
    A. 0—10   B. 10—20
    C. 20—30   D. 30—40
    E. 40—50

72. **The commonest toxic manifestation of impure trilene degradation products is are :**   **AIIMS 1984**
    A. Kidney lesion
    B. Increased intracranial tension
    C. Cranial nerve lesion
    D. Tachypnea

73. **The commonest cranial nerve involved amongst the toxic manifestation of trichloroethylene or its degradation product is :**   **DNB 1991**
    A. 1st   B. 3rd
    C. 5th   D. 7th
    E. 11th

Ans.	57. A	58. B	59. A	60. A	61. A	62. A	63. D	64. D	65. B	66. A
	67. C	68. E	69. C	70. B	71. D	72. C	73. C			

74. The two important impurities caused by decomposition of ether are :   **AMU 1987**
   A. Thymol and dichloroacetylene
   B. Acetic aldehyde and ether peroxide
   C. Alcohol and sulphur dioxide
   D. None of the above

75. All of the following inhalational anaesthetic agents suppress the Hypoxic pulmonary Vasoconstrictor reflex except :   **AMU 1987**
   A. Ether   B. Halothane
   C. Trichloroethylene   D. Nitrous Oxide
   E. Methoxyflurane

76. All are true except one for halothane anaesthesia :   **Bihar 1989**
   A. Increases cerebral blood flow
   B. Raises intracranial pressure
   C. Increases cerebral metabolism
   D. Gastrointestinal motility is decreased

77. Halothane causes all of the following except :   **AIIMS 1988**
   A. Inhibition of sympathetic nervous system
   B. Direct myocardial depression
   C. Central vasomotor depression
   D. Increased vascular resistance

78. The Boiling point of ethylene chloride is :   **AIIMS 1984, 86**
   A. 2.4°C   B. 12.5°
   C. 44°C   D. 79°C

79. Dose of Neostigmine per kg body weight is :   **AIIMS 1984, 85; Delhi 1987, 89**
   A. 0.01 mg/kg   B. 0.1 mg/kg
   C. 1 mg/kg   D. 2 mg/kg

80. Most potent analgesic among following anaesthetics is: **PGI 1985; AMC 1986; Delhi 1987, 88**
   A. Ether   B. Halothane
   C. Trichlorethylene   D. Chloroform

81. High output renal failure may be caused by :   **AIIMS 1986, 87, 89**
   A. Methoxyflurane   B. Diethyl ether
   C. Enflurane   D. Halothane

82. Site of action of muscle relaxants is :   **AIIMS 1988**
   A. Cerebral cortex   B. Reticular formation
   C. Anterior horn cells   D. Myoneural junction

83. Action of which muscle relaxant is prolonged in liver disease :   **AIIMS 1988, 89**
   A. Suxamethonium   B. d-tubocurarine
   C. Gallamine   D. Benzisoquinolium

84. Halothane sensitized the heart to :   **Delhi 1990**
   A. Exogenous epinephrine
   B. Endogenous epinephrine
   C. Dopamine
   D. Anoxia

85. Drug that is used in minimum alveolar concentration is :   **Rajasthan 1994**
   A. Ether   B. Nitrous oxide
   C. Methoxyflurane   D. Cyclopropane

86. The most potent cause of cerebral vasodilation is :   **TN 1990**
   A. Ether   B. Halothane
   C. Barbiturates   D. Increase in PCO_2

87. Disadvantage of N_2O is that :   **AIIMS 1990**
   A. Less efficacy   B. Irritation of mucosa
   C. Less analgesic effect   D. Forms explosive mixture

88. Cerebral Vasoconstriction occurs in anaesthesia by :   **PGI 1994**
   A. Halothane   B. Cyclopropane
   C. Enflurane   D. Isoflurane

89. Match the following :

Agent		Min. Alveolar conc. (volume %)
I.	Nitrous oxide	(i) -33
II.	Methoxyflurane	(ii) 35
III.	Cyclopropane	(iii) -88
IV.	Diethyl ether	(iv) 105
V.	Halothane	(v) 50

   A. I (i)   II (ii)   III (iii)   IV (iv)   V (v)
   B. I (ii)   II (iv)   III (iii)   IV (i)   V (v)
   C. I (iii)   II (iv)   III (i)   IV (ii)   V (v)
   D. I (iv)   II (iii)   III (v)   IV (ii)   V (i)

90. Which is not a feature of non-depolarising blocker :   **PGI 1994**
   A. Flushing   B. Twitching
   C. Prolonged paralysis   D. Respiratory paralysis

91. Regarding the use of halothane in obstetric surgery, which is true :   **C.U.P.G.E.E. 1995**
   A. There is increased risk of PPH
   B. It has no effect on uterine musculature
   C. Best used in caesarean section
   D. None is true

92. N_2O should not be administered in one of the following conditions :   **C.U.P.G.E.E. 1995**
   A. Volvulus of gut
   B. Dental extraction
   C. Obstetric anaesthesia
   D. Wound debridment

Ans.	74. B	75. A	76. C	77. D	78. B	79. A	80. C	81. A	82. D	83. B
	84. B	85. C	86. D	87. A	88. B	89. C	90. B	91. A	92. A	

93. Atracurium is eliminated from the body by :

                                                    PGI 1986
    A. Renal excretion
    B. Hepatic excretion
    C. Both renal and hepatic excretion
    D. Hoffman degradation

94. Shortest acting muscle relaxant is :   AI 1997
    A. Pancuronium   B. Vecuronium
    C. Alcuronium   D. Mivacuronium

95. Prolonged muscle paralysis in a healthy individual may be caused by :

                        Delhi 1981, 83; PGI 1984; ESI 1989
    A. d-tubocurare   B. Gallamine
    C. Pancuronium   D. Succinylcholine

96. In Halothane anaesthesia, depth is best indicated by :
                                                    DNB 1990
    A. BP   B. Respiratory rate
    C. Consciousness   D. Pulse rate

97. In Methoxyflurane use, depth of anaesthesia is best indicated by :   DNB 1989
    A. PR   B. Respiration
    C. BP   D. Pain sensation

98. Methoxyflurane is used in ———% concentration :
                                                    AIIMS 1986
    A. 0.20   B. 0.75
    C. 2.5   D. 3.0

99. Rapid induction by halothane will cause :

                                                    Kerala 1996
    A. Hypotension
    B. Hypertension
    C. Diaphragm paralysis
    D. Central respiratory depression

100. Which of the following does not potentiate d-tubo-curarine :   AIIMS 1981
    A. Halothane   B. Diethyl ether
    C. C_3H_6 D. Ethylene

101. Which of the following is recommended for use in anaesthesia in hyperbaric chambers :   AIIMS 1985
    A. Diethyl ether   B. Cyclopropane
    C. Nitrous oxide   D. Halothane
    E. None of the above

102. The muscle relaxant effect of succinylcholine lasts for:
                                                    AIIMS 1987
    A. 1 minute   B. 2 minutes
    C. 3 to 5 minutes   D. 10 minutes

103. Which of the following occurs first with the use of d-tubocurare :   PGI 1982
    A. Diphragmatic relaxation
    B. Abdominal wall relaxation
    C. Diplopia
    D. Ptosis

104. The muscle which is affected least with d-tubocurare is:
                                                    AIIMS 1983
    A. Facial   B. Diaphragm
    C. Ocular   D. Abdominal

105. Partition coefficient of methoxyflurane is :
                                                    AIIMS 1983
    A. 2.3   B. 13
    C. 15   D. 17

106. Boiling point is minimum of :   AMU 1986
    A. Ether   B. Nitrous oxide
    C. Cyclopropane   D. TCE

107. Features of gallamine include :   AIIMS 1983
    A. Not reversed by neostigmine
    B. Stimulates sympathetic ganglia
    C. Crosses placental barrier
    D. Mostly metabolized in liver

108. Duration of action is minimum of :   DNB 1991
    A. Fazadinium   B. Pancuronium
    C. Vecuronium   D. Atracuronium

109. Fasciculations following injection of succinylcholine are likely to appear first in :   PGI 1982
    A. Hands   B. Eyelids
    C. Legs   D. Abdominal muscles
    E. Chest muscles

110. Metabolites of which of the following is ototoxic :
                                                    DNB 1989
    A. Halothane   B. Methoxyflurane
    C. Cyclopropane   D. TCE

111. Examples of competitive neuromuscular blocking agents include all of the following, except :
                                                    AIIMS 1980
    A. Suxamethonium   B. Gallamine
    C. Tubocurarine   D. Pancuronium

112. The present trend towards the use of nitrous oxide in anaesthesia is :   AIIMS 1982
    A. To use nitrous oxide alone
    B. To use nitrous oxide-oxygen
    C. To use nitrous oxide-oxygen along with small amounts of supplementary anaesthetics
    D. None of the above

113. Abnormalities of the cardiac rhythm are to be expected even in normal individuals with :   PGI 1983
    A. Halothane   B. Cyclopropane
    C. Ether   D. Methoxyflurane

Ans.	93. D	94. D	95. A	96. A	97. B	98. B	99. A	100. D	101. D	102. C
	103. D	104. B	105. B	106. B	107. C	108. C	109. B	110. D	111. A	112. C
	113. B									

114. All are true about trichloroethylene, except :

PGI 1981

A. Should be used in CO_2 absorption systems
B. It is non- inflammable
C. It is non-irritant
D. It may cause tachypnea
E. It decomposes on exposure to light and air

115. Which of the following is most soluble in blood :

AIIMS 1983

A. Nitrous oxide   B. Cyclopropane
C. Halothane   D. Ether
E. All are equally soluble

116. N_2O is contraindicated in :   AMC 1984
A. Pneumothorax   B. Lung of kidney cysts
C. Bronchial fistula   D. All of the above

117. Maintenance of surgical anaesthesia with diethyl ether requires an inhaled concentration of :   AIIMS 1982
A. 1%   B. 2%
C. 3-4%   D. 6-8%
E. 8-12%

118. Halothane (1%) decreases cerebral oxygen utilization by :   PGI 1982
A. 25%   B. 5%
C. 1%   D. 15%
E. None of the above

119. Maintenance of the analgesic stage of ether anaesthesia requires an inhaled concentration of :   AIIMS 1983
A. 1.2%   B. 0.6%
C. 3.4%   D. 3%
E. 5%

120. Muscle relaxant not to be used in liver failure are except :   PGI 1985
A. Pancuronium   B. dTC
C. Suxamethonium   D. Decamethonium

121. Succinylcholine is a muscle relaxant which acts by :

Delhi 1984

A. Persistent depolarisation
B. Competitive blockade
C. Mechanism of action uncertain
D. Both A and B

122. The pin index code for nitrous oxide is :   AIIMS 1987
A. 2, 5   B. 2, 6
C. 1, 6   D. 3, 5
E. 3, 6

123. Which of the following anaesthetics can be self-administered by the patient during labor :   AP 1997
A. Trichloroethylene   B. Ethyl chloride
C. Halothane   D. Enflurane

124. Tachypnea is commonly found in anaesthesia with except :   AIIMS 1980
A. Halothane   B. Cyclopropane
C. Trichloroethylene   D. Diethyl ether

125. Ether is not used in modern surgical practice because :

Kerala 1997

A. Highly explosive
B. Poor anaesthetic
C. Expensive
D. Complicated apparatus needed

126. All of the following contain an ether linkage except :

JIPMER 1998

A. Halothane   B. Isoflurane
C. Methoxy flurane   D. Desflurane

127. Treatment of ether convulsion may include :

UPSC 1983

A. Cooling   B. IV barbiturate
C. Artificial respiration   D. All of the above
E. None of the above

128. Ether decomposition is prevented by :   AIIMS 1982
A. Copper   B. CO_2
C. Both of the above   D. Neither of the above

129. Features of Ketamine "dissociative anaesthesia" include all except :   PGI 1986
A. Profound analgesia
B. Light sleep
C. Increased muscle tone
D. Anaesthesia lasts for about one hour
E. Emergence delirium may occur

130. Physostigmine can reverse the effects of following except: MAHE 1998
A. Amitriptyline   B. Edrophonium
C. d-TC   D. Organophosphates

131. Rapid termination of action of Suxamethonium is due to: MAHE 1998
A. Rapid renal elimination
B. Enzymatic degradation by pseudocholinesterase
C. Metabolised by liver to acetyl CoA
D. Redistribution

132. True about halothane is :

MAHE 1998, 2000; Kerala 1999

A. $\downarrow$ arterial pressure
B. $\uparrow$ HR
C. $\downarrow$ CO
D. $\uparrow$ Sympathoadrenal activity

133. Chloroform decomposes if exposed to :

PGI 1980, 89, 93

A. Light   B. Air
C. Alkalies   D. All of the above
E. None of the above

Ans.	114. A	115. D	116. D	117. A	118. A	119. A	120. D	121. A	122. D	123. A
	124. B	125. A	126. A	127. D	128. A	129. D	130. B	131. B	132. A	133. D

134. Signs of cyclopropane anaesthesia which indicate that anaesthesia is too deep except :
     Delhi 1983 ; AIIMS 1986
     A. Ventricular ectopic beats
     B. Heart rate below 50/min
     C. Hypotension unrelated to surgery or haemorrhage
     D. Laryngospam
     E. None of the above

135. Depolarising agents have associated with all of the following, except :   **AP 1995**
     A. Muscle fasciculations preceding the onset of block.
     B. Absence of post-tetanic potentiation.
     C. Potentiation of block by anticholinesterases.
     D. Reversal by anticholinesterases.

136. The concentration of halothane which can cause death is :   **Rajasthan 1993**
     A. 10 mg%   B. 20 mg%
     C. 60 mg%   D. 180 mg%

137. Post-anaesthetic muscle pain is caused by :
     AIIMS 1993
     A. d TC   B. Gallamine
     C. Suxamethonium   D. Xylocaine

138. In myaesthenia gravis, which of the following is true about sensitivity to curare and scoline :   **AIIMS 1994**

	Curare	Scoline
A.	Increased	Decreased
B.	Decreased	Increased
C.	Increased	Increased
D.	Decreased	Normal

139. Shortest acting non-depolarizing anaesthetic agent is :
     AIIMS 1984; Delhi 1994
     A. Atracurium   B. Vecuronium
     C. d-TC   D. Scoline

140. All are true about nitrous oxide except :   **Kerala 1999**
     A. Megaloblastic anemia
     B. Bone marrow depression
     C. Causes teratogenicity
     D. Safe in middle ear surgery

141. Which of the following does not cause ↑ICT :
     Delhi 2000
     A. Halothane   B. Ketamine
     C. Isoflurane   D. Enflurane

142. Highest MAC is of :   **Delhi 2000**
     A. N₂O   B. Enflurane
     C. Halothane   D. Desflurane

143. During reversal of Anaesthesia the drugs commonly used are :   **TNPSC 1995**
     A. D-Tubocurarine

B. Neostigmine and Atropine
C. Scoline
D. Adrenaline or non-adrenaline

144. **Assertion (A) :** Atracurium is the ideal muscle relaxant in renal failure.
     Reason (R) : It is neither broken down nor excreted by the kidney.   **TNPSC 1995**
     A. Both (A) and (R) are correct and (R) is the correct explanation.
     B. (A) alone is true and (R) is false.
     C. (A) is false and (R) is true.
     D. Both (A) and (R) are true but (R) is not a correct explanation.

145. Suxamethonium is contraindicated in all except :
     UP 2000
     A. Pre-operative hypokalemia
     B. Pre-operative hyperkalemia
     C. Open eye surgery
     D. Paraplegia

146. A man with alcoholic lever failure requires general anaesthesia for surgery. Anaesthetic agent of choice is :
     AI 2001
     A. Ether   B. Halothane
     C. Methoxyflurane D. Isoflurane

147. All of the following are true except :   **AI 2001**
     A. Halothane is a good analgesic
     B. Halothane sensitise the heart for catecholamines
     C. Halothane causes liver damage
     D. Hypotension is common

148. Propofol is used as IV induction agent in total intravenous anaesthesia as :   **JIPMER 2002**
     A. It does not reduce arterial pressure
     B. It doesn't cause respiratory depression
     C. Doesn't affect renal function
     D. Recovery is rapid even if used for long time

149. Which of the following inhibits hypoxic pulmonary vasoconstriction in a dose related fashion : **Delhi 2001**
     A. Halothane   B. Ketamine
     C. Propofol   D. Thiopentone

150. Which muscle relaxant increases intracranial pressure:
     AIIMS 2002
     A. Mivacurium   B. Atracurium
     C. Suxamethonium   D. Vecuronium

151. The use of succinylcholine is not contraindicated in :
     AIIMS 2002
     A. Tetanus   B. Closed head injury
     C. Cerebral stroke D. Hepatic failure

Ans.	134. D	135. D	136. B	137. B	138. A	139. D	140. C	141. D	142. A	143. B
	144. A	145. A	146. D	147. A	148. D	149. A	150. C	151. C		

152. A 6-years old boy is scheduled for examination of the eye under anaesthesia. The father informed that for the past six months the child is developing progressive weakness of both legs. His elder sibling had died at the age of 14 years. Which drug would you definitely avoid during the anaesthetic management :
                                                    AIIMS 2002
   A. Succinylcholine   B. Thiopentone
   C. Nitrous oxide   D. Vecuronium

153. Which of the following statement is not correct for vancuronium :   AIIMS 2002
   A. It has high incidence of cardiovascular side effects.
   B. It has short duration of neuromuscular block.
   C. In usual doses the dose adjustment is not required in kidney disease.
   D. It has high liphophilic property.

154. At the end of a balanced anaesthesia technique with non-depolarising muscle relaxant, a patient recovered spontaneously from the effect of muscle relaxant without any reversal. Which is the most probable relaxant the patient had received :   AI 2003
   A. Pancuronium   B. Gallamine
   C. Atracurium   D. Vecuronium

Ans.   152. A   153 C   154. C

EXPLANATIONS OF AGENTS & MUSCLE RELAXANTS

1.   Ans. — D.   Succinylcholine

2.   Ans. — D.   Increased heart rate secondary to a decrease in total peripheral resistance.

Cardiac output is decreased by halothane secondary to bradycardia, an effect reversed by atropine.

3.   Ans. — D.   All of the above

4.   Ans. — A.   60%

5.   Ans. — D.   The presence of post-tetanic facilitation.

6.   Ans. — D.   Ketamine

7.   Ans. — D.   Diffusion hypoxia

8.   Ans. — B.   Ethylene oxide

9.   Ans. — D.   Gallamine

10. Ans. — B.   Dantrolene

11. Ans. — B.   Halothane

12. Ans. — B.   Halothane

13. Ans. — B.   Malignant hypertension

14. Ans. — C.   Gallamine

They are sensitive to Curare and Gallamine and resistant to suxamethonium. Muscle relaxants should not be used. If anaesthesia is required, use local anaesthesia and if GA is required, use N_2O and Halothane or Enflurane.

15. Ans. — C.   Diethyl Ether

Cyclopropane and Enflurane also sensitizes heart to catecholamines unlike Ether, Fluroxene, and Isoflurane.

16. Ans. — B.   Ketamine

17. Ans. — C.   Halothane

18. Ans. — C.   Methoxyflurane

19. Ans. — D.   Atracuronium

20. Ans. — A.   Halothane

21. Ans. — A.   Ketamine

22. Ans. — A.   Eyelids

23. Ans. — D. N_2O

24. Ans. — A.   Gallamine

Gallamine is contraindicated in presence of CRF. Alcuronium, Pancuronium or dTC can be used. Decamethonium and Gallamine are excreted unchanged through kidney and crosses placental barrier unlike d-TC.

25. Ans. — B.   500 mg

26. Ans. — A.   Trilene

27. Ans. — C.   75%

28. Ans. — B.   Ethylchloride

29. Ans. — D.   Kanamycin

Streptomycin, Kanamycin and other aminoglycosides and also Tetracyclines, Clindamycin and lincomycin, calcium channel blockers synergizes the muscle relaxation effects of competitive blockers.

30. Ans. — B.   Heavier than air

Cyclopropane or trimethylene is stored in orange cylinders as a liquid at a pressure of 5 bar no reducing valves being required. It was first synthesized by August von Freund (1835-1892). Its anaesthetic properties were shown by W.H. Lucas and V.E. Henderson and used on a human volunteer by W. Easson Brown, the patient being Professor Henderson.

31. Ans. — C.   Burns

32. Ans. — D.   Causes the expansion of air filled body cavities.

33. Ans. — B.   Sf6

N_2O is a good analgesic agent used commonly in dentistry and in management of post-operative pain.

34. Ans.— A. Methyoxyflurane

Blood gas coefficient of Methyoxyflurane is 13. Cyclopropane has blood gas coefficient of 10. Ether has 12 and Isoflurane 1.4. Read physical and anaesthetic properties of inhalational anaesthetics from Table in K.D. Tripathi's Essentials of Medical Pharmacology.

35. Ans.— D. Trilene
36. Ans.— C. Isoflurane
37. Ans.— D. Diethylether
38. Ans.— D. Femoral vein
39. Ans.— A. Neostigmine may reverse the neuromuscular blockade.
40. Ans.— B. Halothane
41. Ans.— D. Halothane
42. Ans.— D. Both B and C are true
43. Ans.— D. All of the above
44. Ans.— D. All of the above
45. Ans.— B. Cyclopropane
46. Ans.— D. All of the above
47. Ans.— D. Diaphragm
48. Ans.— A. 3 months to 3 years old
49. Ans.— A. Nitrous oxide
50. Ans.— C. Gallamine
51. Ans.— A. Halothane
52. Ans.— D. Ephedrine
53. Ans.— C. Muscle relaxant
54. Ans.— A. Competitive block of nicotinic receptor
55. Ans.— A. Halothane
56. Ans.— B. Neostigmine
57. Ans.— A. d-tubocurarine
58. Ans.— B. Nitrous oxide is in gaseous form in the cylinder.
59. Ans.— A. Halothane
60. Ans.— A. Ether

Insulin need of a diabetic is increased with ether GA. Switch over to plain insulin even if the patient is on oral hypoglycemics.

61. Ans.— A. N_2O

Immediately after nitrous oxide anaesthesia, hypoxia may occur because it diffuses out into alveolar space faster than nitrogen can diffuse in. The dilution of alveolar oxygen causes diffusion hypoxia. Oxygen should be given during first 10-15 min after anaesthesia.

62. Ans.— A. Trilene
63. Ans.— D. All of the above
64. Ans.— D. All of the above
65. Ans.— B. Neostigmine methyl sulphate
66. Ans.— A. -7°C
67. Ans.— C. Use of large doses of suxamethonium
68. Ans.— E. All of the above
69. Ans.— C. Bronchial Asthma
70. Ans.— B. Provide Good Muscular Relaxation
71. Ans.— D. 30—40
72. Ans.— C. Cranial nerve lesion
73. Ans.— C. 5th
74. Ans.— B. Acetic aldehyde and ether peroxide
75. Ans.— A. Ether
76. Ans.— C. Increases cerebral metabolism
77. Ans.— D. Increased vascular resistance

It decreases vascular resistance and causes hypotension.

78. Ans.— B. 12.5°
79. Ans.— A. 0.01 mg/kg
80. Ans.— C. Trichloroethylene
81. Ans.— A. Methoxyflurane
82. Ans.— D. Myoneural junction
83. Ans.— B. d-tubocurarine
84. Ans.— B. Endogenous epinephrine
85. Ans.— C. Methoxyflurane
86. Ans.— D. Increase in PCO_2
87. Ans.— A. Less efficacy
88. Ans.— B. Cyclopropane
89. Ans.— C. I (iii) II (iv) III (i)   IV (ii) V (v)
90. Ans.— B. Twitching
91. Ans.— A. There is increased risk of PPH
92. Ans.— A. Volvulus of gut
93. Ans.— D. Hoffman degradation

It is eliminated by Hoffman degradation and alkaline ester hydrolysis.

94. Ans.— D. Mivacuronium
95. Ans.— A. d-tubocurare
96. Ans.— A. BP
97. Ans.— B. Respiration
98. Ans.— B. 0.75
99. Ans.— A. Hypotension
100. Ans.— D. Ethylene

101. Ans. — D. Halothane

102. Ans. — C. 3 to 5 minutes

103. Ans. — D. Ptosis

104. Ans. — B. Diaphragm

d-TC causes flaccid paralysis, first on small muscles (fingers, extraocular) hands, feet, arms, leg, neck, face-trunk-intercostal muscles-diaphragm.

105. Ans. — B. 13

106. Ans. — B. Nitrous oxide

107. Ans. — C. Crosses placental barrier

108. Ans. — C. Vecuronium

109. Ans. — B. Eyelids

110. Ans. — D. TCE

111. Ans. — A. Suxamethonium

112. Ans. — C. To use nitrous oxide-oxygen along with small amounts of supplementary anaesthetics.

113. Ans. — B. Cyclopropane

114. Ans. — A. Should be used in CO_2 absorption systems.

115. Ans. — D. Ether

116. Ans. — D. All of the above

117. Ans. — A. 1%

118. Ans. — A. 25%

119. Ans. — A. 1.2%

120. Ans. — D. Decamethonium

121. Ans. — A. Persistent depolarisation

122. Ans. — D. 3, 5

123. Ans. — A. Trichloroethylene

124. Ans. — B. Cyclopropane

125. Ans. — A. Highly explosive

126. Ans. — A. Halothane

127. Ans. — D. All of the above

128. Ans. — A. Copper

129. Ans. — D. Anaesthesia lasts for about one hour

130. Ans. — B. Edrophonium

131. Ans. — B. Enzymatic degradation by pseudocholinesterase.

132. Ans. — A. ↓ arterial pressure

133. Ans. — D. All of the above

134. Ans. — D. Laryngospam

135. Ans. — D. Reversal by anticholinesterases

136. Ans. — B. 20 mg%

137. Ans. — B. Gallamine

It is due to twitching before causing paralysis. Many methods have been advocated to reduce it but non is wholly satisfactory. It also increases IOP and ICP (unlike-TC).

138. Ans. — A. Increased   Decreased

139. Ans. — D. Scoline

140. Ans. — C. Causes teratogenicity

141. Ans. — D. Enflurane

142. Ans. — A. N_2O

MAC of N_2O is 105 and those of Halothane is 0.75, Enflurane 1.68 and Desflurane is 6.0.

143. Ans. — B. Neostigmine and Atropine

144. Ans. — A. Both (A) and (R) are correct and (R) is the correct explanation.

145. Ans. — A. Pre-operative hypokalemia

146. Ans. — D. Isoflurane

Halothane is contraindicated because Halothane is a cumulative drug and cause hepatitis and hepatic necrosis. The other anaesthetic drugs may aggravate this.

147. Ans. — A. Halothane is a good analgesic.

148. Ans. — D. Recovery is rapid even if used for long time.

149. Ans. — A. Halothane

150. Ans. — C. Suxamethonium

151. Ans. — C. Cerebral stroke

152. Ans. — A. Succinylcholine

153. Ans. — C. In usual doses the dose adjustment is not required in kidney disease.

154. Ans. — C. Atracurium

* Recovery index time of Atracurium is 13 minutes in Adults and 10 minutes in children.

4-D. MCQ's OF MISCELLANEOUS ASPECTS OF G. A.

1. **Biphasic respiratory depression is usually seen after :**
    AMU 1988, 92
    A. Neuroleptanaesthesia   B. Regional anaesthesia
    C. Halothane anaesthesia   D. Isoflurane anaesthesia

2. **In the presence of pneumocephalus created either by surgery or by performance of a pneumoencephalogram, it is suggested that nitrous oxide be avoided for how many days :**   **AIIMS 1986**
    A. 4 days   B. 5 days
    C. 6 days   D. 7 days
    E. 10 days

3. **Anaesthetic agent associated with hallucination is :**
    AIIMS 1992, 94, 95, 99, 2002
    A. Ketamine   B. Halothane
    C. Ether   D. Cyclopropane

4. **Anaesthetic which increases myocardial oxygen demand is :**   **PGI 1993, 97**
    A. Ketamine   B. Halothane
    C. Enflurane   D. Ether

5. **I.V. anaesthetic agent causing maximum bronchodilation is :**   **JIPMER 1993; Rajasthan 1998**
    A. Ketamine   B. Halothane
    C. Thiopentone   D. Fentanyl

6. **Histamine is released by all except :**   **Delhi 1993**
    A. d-TC   B. Succinylcholine
    C. Morphine   D. Pentamidine

7. **Maximum interior relaxation is seen with :**
    Delhi 1992
    A. Ether   B. Halothane
    C. Spinal anaesthesia   D. Trilene

8. **In the presence of (Beta) blockade agents anaesthetic agents that produce myocardial depression is/are :**
    DNB 1990
    A. Ether   B. Cyclopropane
    C. Trichloroethylene   D. Only A and B are true
    E. Only B and C are true

9. **Muscle rigidity is increased with the use of :**
    AIIMS 1990
    A. Physostigmine   B. Neostigmine
    C. Fentanyl   D. Droperidol

10. **'Sea saw' respiration is characteristic of :**   **DNB 1990**
    A. Respiratory obstruction   B. Partial curarization
    C. Deep after anaesthesia   D. All of the above
    E. None of the above

11. **Least cardiotoxic anaesthetic agent is :**   **AI 1996, 98**
    A. Enflurane   B. Isoflurane
    C. TCE   D. Halothane

12. **Which of the following crosses the blood brain barrier :**
    AP 1989
    A. Halothane   B. Thiopentone
    C. Glycopyrollate   D. Cyclopropane

13. **Hypotension in anaesthesia can be induced by all of the following drugs except :**   **DNB 1990**
    A. Pancuronium   B. Halothane
    C. Hexamethonium   D. Sodium nitroprusside

14. **Which anaesthetic is used in surgery on patients with hepatorenal failure :**   **PGI 1994**
    A. Gallamine   B. Atracuronium
    C. Pancuronium   D. d-TC

15. **Liver Cell necrosis can occur due to :**
    AIIMS 1984; Kerala 1990
    A. Digoxin   B. Gallamine
    C. Halothane   D. Ether

16. **Malignant hyperthermia is seen with following, except :**   **PGI 1995**
    A. Halothane   B. Enflurane
    C. Isoflurane   D. N_2O

17. **In status asthmaticus, the anaesthetic agent used as bronchodilator is :**   **AIIMS 1984**
    A. Morphine   B. Thiopentone sodium
    C. Ketamine   D. Halothane

18. **Use of which drug during anaesthesia may cause muscle spasm :**   **UP 1996**
    A. Physostigmine   B. Buprenorphine
    C. Fentanyl   D. D-tubocurare

Ans.	1. A	2. D	3. A	4. A	5. A	6. D	7. A	8. D	9. D	10. D
	11. B	12. B	13. A	14. B	15. C	16. D	17. C	18. C		

19. In acute intermittent porphyria, one can use :
    Delhi 1984
    A. Thiopentone   B. Methohexiotone
    C. Propanidid   D. None

20. Maximum fluoride ions are provided by :   **Delhi 1990**
    A. Isofluorane   B. Enflurane
    C. Methoxyfluorane   D. Cyclopropane

21. Excessive salivation is produced by :   **Delhi 1983**
    A. Ketamine   B. Thiopentone
    C. Suxamethonium   D. Diazepam

22. The most efficient respiratory stimulant is :
    AIIMS 1982
    A. Nikethamide   B. Amiphenazole
    C. Pretheamide   D. Doxapram

23. In Day case surgery, anaesthesia of choice is :
    AIIMS 1998
    A. Propofol   B. Thiopentone
    C. Halothane   D. Diazepam

24. Bone marrow depression is seen with :   **AIIMS 1995**
    A. N_2O B. Halothane
    C. Isoflurane   D. Ether

25. Bandle's contraction ring is most rapidly treated by :
    AIIMS 1982
    A. Succinyl choline   B. Halothane
    C. Spinal anaesthesia   D. d-Tubocurarine
    E. Incision

26. Which of the following causes bronchodilation by central action on respiratory centre :   **AIIMS 1981**
    A. Pentothal sodium   B. Paraldehyde
    C. Tribromethanol   D. Cyclopropane
    E. None of the above

27. Early signs of exhaustion of sodalime include :
    PGI 1983
    A. Shallow respiration   B. Rate in blood pressure
    C. Fall in pulse-rate   D. Hypotension
    E. Decreased cozing

28. Inhalation of a gas mixture containing which anaesthetic agent at a partial pressure of 30 Torr will produce rapid anaesthesia :   **PGI 1984**
    A. Nitrous oxide   B. Cyclopropane
    C. Halothane   D. Ether
    E. None of the above

29. Malignant hyperthermia is best treated with :
    AIIMS 1987
    A. Dantrolene sodium   B. Pottasium chloride
    C. Atropine   D. Corticosteroids

30. The anaesthetic that effects the Laryngeal & Pharyngeal reflexes minimally :   **AP 1997**
    A. Propanidid   B. Methohexitone
    C. Thiopentone   D. Ketamine

31. Least fluoride content is present in :   **PGI 1997**
    A. Methoxyflurane   B. Enflurane
    C. Isoflurane   D. Sevoflurane

32. Stage-I, Plane 2 is reached in anaesthesia when there is:
    Karnataka 1989
    A. Total analgesia-total amnesia-loss of consciousness
    B. Loss of lid reflex
    C. Partial analgesia-pre-amnesia
    D. Partial analgesia-total amnesia

33. In raised ICT, following anaesthetic agent is used :
    AIIMS 1994
    A. Enflurane   B. Halothane
    C. TCE   D. N_2O

34. Which of the following is contraindicated in epilepsy :
    AIIMS 1994
    A. Enflurane   B. Isoflurane
    C. Isoflurane   D. Ether

35. Safe anaesthesia in a child is :   **Delhi 1994**
    A. Halothane   B. Enflurane
    C. Methoxyflurane   D. Ether

36. Which is not an intravenous anaesthetic :   **AI 1995**
    A. Etomidate   B. Thiopentone
    C. Ketamine   D. Cyclopropane

37. Post-spinal headache is due to :   **AI 1995**
    A. Injury to spinal cord   B. CSF leak from dura
    C. Meningitis   D. Meningism

38. Best way to prevent hypotension during spinal anaesthesia is :   **AI 1995**
    A. Preloading with crystalloids
    B. Dopamine
    C. Mephenteramine
    D. Trendelenburg's position

Match the following (Ques. 39 to 42):
    AIIMS 1983; Delhi 1984

Colour of cylinder   *Gas*
39. Blue   A. Carbon dioxide
40. Grey   B. Nitrous oxide
41. Black body with   C. Cyclopropane
    white top
42. Orange   D. Oxygen

Match the following (Ques. 43 to 46):
    AIIMS 1986

43. Oxygen   A. 750 pound per square inch
44. Nitrous oxide   B. 75 pound per square inch
45. Cyclopropane   C. 2000 pound per square inch
46. Carbon Dioxide   D. 50 pound per square inch

Ans.	19. C	20. C	21. A	22. D	23. A	24. C	25. B	26. C	27. B	28. C
	29. A	30. D	31. A	32. C	33. D	34. A	35. D	36. D	37. B	38. A
	39. B	40. A	41. D	42. C	43. C	44. A	45. B	46. D		

W.47. The rate of induction of anaesthesia by an inhalational agent is increased by a : Karnataka 1999

A. High alveolar ventilation rate
B. High partial pressure of anaesthetic in inspired air
C. High tissue/gas solubility coefficient
D. Low body mass

48. Which of the following reduces intracranial tension : Kerala 1999

A. Ketamine
B. Enflurane
C. Halothane
D. Phenobarbitone

49. Which of the following is correctly matched : TNPSC 1998

A. Gallamine-Kidney
B. Suxamethonium-Liver & Kidney
C. Atracurium-Pseudo-Cholinesterase
D. Vecuronium-Hoffman degradation

50. In bronchial asthma, anaesthesia of choice is : AIIMS 2000

A. Propanidid
B. Ketamine
C. Althesin
D. Thiopentone

51. Unpleasant dreams and aggressive violence are associated with the use of which of the following anaesthetic agents : Kerala 2000

A. Ketamine hydrochloride
B. Thiopentone sodium
C. Propofol
D. Etomidate
E. Methohexitone

52. What is the critical concentration of serum inorganic fluoride, which when exceeded results in nephrotoxicity consistently : Kerala 2000

A. $50\,\mu M$ per litre
B. $30\,\mu M$ per litre
C. $20\,\mu M$ per litre
D. $10\,\mu M$ per litre
E. $5\,\mu M$ per litre

53. Which of the anaesthetic agent is maximally metabolized : Kerala 2001

A. Methoxyflurane
B. Halothane
C. Nitrous oxide
D. Isoflurane

54. Sudden decrease in end tidal CO_2 under general anaesthesia suggests : Delhi 2001

A. Hypothermia
B. Malignant hyperpyrexia
C. Cardiac arrest
D. Accidental extubation

55. Rapid induction of anaesthesia occurs with which of the following inhalational anaesthetics : AIIMS 2002

A. Isoflurane
B. Halothane
C. Desflurane
D. Sevoflurane

56. The m opoid receptor is responsible for the following effects except : AIIMS 2002

A. Miosis
B. Bradycardia
C. Hypothermia
D. Bronchodilation

57. Which of the following inhaled gas is used to decrease pulmonary artery pressure in adults and infants : AIIMS 2002

A. 6-mereaptopurine
B. Vincristine
C. Bleomycin
D. Adriamycin

58. During rapid sequence induction of anaesthesia : AI 2003

A. Sellick's manoeuver is not required.
B. Pre-oxygenation is mandatory.
C. Suxamethonium is contraindicated.
D. Patient is mechanically ventilated before endotracheal intubation.

59. Which of the following is the best indication for propofol as an intravenous induction agent: AI 2004

A. Neurosurgery
B. Day care surgery
C. Patients with coronary artery disease
D. In neonates

60. Which of the following volatile anaesthetic agents should be preferred for induction of anaesthesia in children: AI 2004

A. Enflurane
B. Isoflurane
C. Sevoflurane
D. Desflurane

61. When a patient develops supraventricular tachycardia with hypotension under general anaesthesia, all of the following treatments may be instituted except: AI 2004

A. Carotid sinus massage
B. Adenosine 3–12 mg IV
C. Direct current cardioversion
D. Verapamil 5 mg IV

62. Which one of the following is the fastest acting inhalational agent? AI 2005

A. Halothane
B. Isoflurane
C. Ether
D. Sevoflurane

63. All of the following are the disadvantages of anaesthetic ether, except : AI 2005

A. Induction is slow.
B. Irritant nature of ether increases salivary and bronchial secretions.
C. Cautery can not be used.
D. Affects blood pressure and is liable to produce arrhythmias.

Ans.	47. ALL	48. D	49. A	50. B	51. A	52. A	53. A	54. D	55. C	56. D
	57. C	58. B	59. B	60. C	61. A	62. D	63. D			

EXPLANATIONS OF MISCELLANEOUS ASPECTS OF G.A.

1.   Ans. — A.   Neuroleptanaesthesia

2.   Ans. — D.   7 days

3.   Ans. — A.   Ketamine

This is reduced by lorazepam premedication and allowing the patient to rest in a quiet room.

4.   Ans. — A.   Ketamine

5.   Ans. — A.   Ketamine

6.   Ans. — D.   Pentamidine

7.   Ans. — A.   Ether

8.   Ans. — D.   Only A and B are true

9.   Ans. — D.   Droperidol

10. Ans. — D.   All of the above

11. Ans. — B.   Isoflurane

Isoflurane does not sensitize heart to catecholamines and give stability to cardiac rhythm, Enflurane and halothane are myocardial depressants.

12. Ans. — B.   Thiopentone

13. Ans. — A.   Pancuronium

14. Ans. — B.   Atracuronium

15. Ans. — C.   Halothane

16. Ans. — D. N_2O

17. Ans. — C.   Ketamine

18. Ans. — C.   Fentanyl

19. Ans. — C.   Propanidid

20. Ans. — C.   Methoxyfluorane

21. Ans. — A.   Ketamine

22. Ans. — D.   Doxapram

23. Ans. — A.   Propofol

24. Ans. — C.   Isoflurane

Never use it alone in subjects with severe cardiac or pulmonary disease or anaemia or in young children. Prolonged use is seen in Polio and tetanus.

25. Ans. — B.   Halothane

26. Ans. — C.   Tribromethanol

27. Ans. — B.   Rate in blood pressure

28. Ans. — C.   Halothane

29. Ans. — A.   Dantrolene sodium

30. Ans. — D.   Ketamine

31. Ans. — A.   Methoxyflurane

32. Ans. — C.   Partial analgesia-pre-amnesia

33. Ans. — D. N_2O

34. Ans. — A.   Enflurane

35. Ans. — D.   Ether

Morphine is not used in children because special care is necessary on infants under 6 months aged, feeble and debilitated and patients with a raised pCO_2, suprarenal insufficiency, myasthenia, myotonia, hypothyroidism, asthma, raised ICT, respiratory depression, hepatic or renal failure, acute alcoholism, diverticulitis and labour. It kills by causing respiratory arrest.

36. Ans. — D.   Cyclopropane

Cyclopropane is an inhalational anaesthetic.

37. Ans. — B.   CSF leak from dura

Other methods which may help are lying down of the patient with foot end of bed raised, in semidarkness about 6 hours after operation. Reading and smoking prohibited for a further six hours. The administration of codeine or pethidine is helpful and patient should be encouraged to drink as much as possible.

38. Ans. — A.   Preloading with crystalloids

Hypotension is below 80-90 mmHg systolic.

39. Ans. — B.   Nitrous oxide

N_2O has blue coloured cylinder, O_2 black with white top CO_2- grey and Cyclopropane (orange). Combinations of these standard colours.

40.   Ans.— A.   Carbon dioxide
41.   Ans.— D.   Oxygen
42.   Ans.— C.   Cyclopropane
43.   Ans.— C.   2000 pound per square inch
44.   Ans.— A.   750 pound per square inch
45.   Ans.— B.   75 pound per square inch
46.   Ans.— D.   50 pound per square inch
47.   Ans.— B.   ALL
48.   Ans.— D.   Phenobarbitone
49.   Ans.— A.   Gallamine-Kidney
50.   Ans.— B.   Ketamine
51.   Ans.— A.   Ketamine hydrochloride
52.   Ans.— A.   50 m M per litre
53.   Ans.— A.   Methoxyflurane
54.   Ans.— D.   Accidental extubation
55.   Ans.— C.   Desflurane
56.   Ans.— D.   Bronchodilation
57.   Ans.— C.   Bleomycin
58.   Ans.— B.   Pre-oxygenation is mandatory

      *   The technique to induce Anaesthesia followed almost by tracheal intubation (so-called crash induction) is designed to prevent the dangers of vomiting, regurgitation & aspiration of stomach contents. It is done under control of suxamethonium (fast acting muscle relaxant).

      Note : Pre-oxigenation is not necessary.

59.   Ans.— B.   Day care surgery

      Propofol :

      •   It is an oily liquid employed as a 1% emulsion for I.V. induction and short duration anaesthesia.

      •   It lacks airway irritancy and is particularly suited for outpatient surgery because residual impairment is less marked and incidence of post-operative nausea and vomiting is low.

      •   Intermittent injection or continuous infusion of propofol has been used for total I.V. anaesthesia when supplemented by fentanyl.

60.   Ans.— C.   Sevoflurane

      Sevoflurane allowing smooth induction of anaesthesia in infants and children.

      Sevoflurane :

      •   Unlike desflurane, it poses no problem in induction; acceptability is good even by pediatric patients.

      •   It is likely to become popular both for outpatient as well as inpatient surgery.

      •   It does not cause sympathetic stimulation and airway irritation even during rapid induction.

      Isoflurane :

      •   It has an irritant, etheral odour that is associated with an increased incidence of airway problems such as coughing and laryngospasm during induction, maintenance and recovery from anaesthesia.

      Desflurane :

      •   Like isoflurane, it has a markedly pungent etheral odour, making it unsuitable for inhalation induction of anaesthesia in children.

61.   Ans.— A.   Carotid sinus massage

      Supraventricular tachycardia :

      •   In patients without hypotension, vagal manoeuvers, particularly carotid sinus massage, can't terminate the arrhythmia in 80% of cases.

      •   Verapamid (2.5 to 10 mg IV) or adenosine (6-12 mg. IV) is the agent of choice.

      •   If severe ischemia and/or hypotension is caused by the tachycardia, DC cardioversion should be considered.

62.   Ans.— D.   Sevoflurane

      Blood Gas Co-efficient-decides whether any agent will have fast induction, change of depth and recovery or slow.

      The lower the value the faster will be the agent.

      Now let's see Blood gas coefficient of few agents :

Agent	B/G Coefficient
Desflurane	0.42
Nitrous Oxide	0.47
Sevoflurane	0.67
Isoflurane	1.4
Enflurane	1.9
Halothane	2.3
Ether	12

      So, out of the given choices Sevoflurane has the lowest B/G coefficient hence is the fastest.

63.   Ans. — D.   Affects blood pressure and is liable to produce arrhythmias :

Ether :

* Ether blood/gas partition coefficient 12.0.
* Slow induction and recovery.
* Minimum alveolar concentration 1.92.
* Flammable in air and explosive in O_2.
* *Irritant vapour, which can readily induce laryngeal spasm and make induction even slower.*
* Ether stimulates alivary and bronchial secretions and so atropine premedication is given.
* Muscle relaxants need not to be used as either itself produces excellent relaxation.

* Ether liberates catecholamines and tends to maintain blood pressure.
* There is little cardiac depression.
* Dysrhythmias are rare.
* Adrenaline is relatively safe with ether.
* Bronchial smooth muscle is relaxed.
* The products of its metabolism (alcohol, acetaldehyde and acetic acid) are relatively non-toxic.
* It should not be used when diathermy is needed in the airways, because of the risk of the fire or explosion, although these have not occurred when air is used to carry the ether vapour.

5

IMPORTANT TEXT OF MISCELLANEOUS

ANATOMICAL CAUSES OF DIFFICULT INTUBATION

1. A short muscular neck and full set of teeth.
2. Receding lower jaw with obtuse mandibular angles.
3. Protruding incisors with relative outgrowth of the premaxilla.
4. Long high arched palate with a long narrow mouth.
5. Increased alveolar-mental distance requiring wide opening of the mandible for laryngoscopy.
6. Poor mobility of the mandible.
7. Increase in posterior depth of the mandible hindering displacement of the mandible.
8. Decreased distance between the occiput and the spinous process of C.

COMMON CAUSES OF PNEUMOTHORAX DURING ANAESTHESIA

Traumatic	Chest injury	
	Rib fracture	
Iatrogenic	Subclavian cannulae	Cervical surgery
	Internal jugular cannulae	Thoracic surgery
	Brachial plexus block	
	Inadvertent barotrauma	
Spontaneous	Localized disorder e.g.	Congenital bullae
	Marfan's syndrome	
	Generalized emphysema	
	Secondary to lung disease abscess	
	Spontaneous mediastinal emphysema	
	Asthma	
	Rapid decompression of livers	

COMMON CAUSES OF ARRYTHMIA DURING ANAESTHESIA

Surgical	Ophthalmic
	Nasal Surgery
	Dental
	Mesenteric traetion
	Anal stretch
Metabolic	Hyperthyroidism
	Hypercapnia
	Hypokalemia
Disease	Congenital heart disease
	Ischemic heart disease
Drugs	Atropine
	Adrenaline
	Halothane
	Cyclopropane

SURGICAL AND OTHER CAUSES OF AIR EMBOLISM

Neurosurgery	Posterior fossa operations in sitting position
Abdominal surgery	Laparoscopy
	Hysterectomy
	D&C and insufflation
Orthopaedic surgery	Arthrography
	Hip surgery
Chest	Open heart surgery
	Breast surgery
Miscellaneous	Middle ear surgery
	Neck surgery
	Blood transfusion
	CVP lines
	Pressure at depth
	Arterial monitoring
	Extradural injection

DRUGS TO BE AVOIDED IN SURGERY FOR PHEOCHROMOCYTOMA

Atropine	Cyclopropane
Suxamethonium	Diethylether
Gallamine	TCE
d-TC	Intra/Extradural blocking agents

Preperative treatment of Pheochromocytoma

Sodium nitroprusside	Most useful to control hypertension pre-operatively
β adrenergic blockage or lignocaine	required to control serious arrythmias
	Neuroleptic followed by normocapnic IPPV using
Induction	Atracuruim or vecuronium for muscle relaxation and an opioid for analgesic supplementation.

MANAGEMENT OF IMPORTANT ARRHYTHMIAS DURING CPR

Arrhythmia	Significance	Treatment
Ventricular fibrillation	No cardiac output Lignocaine if recurrent	DC shock 200 J
Ventricular tachycardia	Cardiac output ↓ or absent, may precipitate VF	If cardiac output reasonable, lignocaine. If pulseless, DC shock 200 J
Ventricular ectopics	May herald VF/VT if frequent, multi-focal or R-on-T	Suppress with lignocaine
Complete heart block	May cause profound hypotension or herald asystole	Isoprenaline infusion until transvenous pacemaker in situ
2°Heart block Mobitz type-II	May progress to complete block	Transvenous pacemeker

(Contd....)

MANAGEMENT OF IMPORTANT ARRHYTHMIAS DURING CPR (Contd...)

Arrhythmia	Significance	Treatment
Artrial fibrillation	Cardiac output ↓ from	1. Synchronised DC shock 50 J if patient deteriorating
Artrial flutter	1. Loss of artrial contraction 2. Fast ventricular rate	2. Digitalisation 3. Practolol
Supraventricular tachycardia	As artrial fibrillation	1. Carotid sinus massage 2. Synchronised DC shock 50 J if patient deteriorating 3. Digitalisation 4. Practolol
Asystole	No cardiac output	Adrenaline Calcium chloride Pacing

Note: Adrenaline, lignocaine and atropine are rapidly effective intratracheally if diluted to 10 ml volume.

CAUSES OF POST-OPERATIVE HYPOVENTILATION

Factors affecting airway	Factors affecting respiratory drive	Peripheral factors
Upper airway obstruction: 　tongue 　laryngospasm 　oedema, foreign body 　tumor	Respiratory depressant drugs Pre-operative CNS pathology Intra or post-operative CVA, Hypothermia	Muscle weakness residual Pre-operative NM disease Electrolyte abnormalities
Bronchospasm	Recent hyperventilation (Pa CO_2 low)	Pain Distension Obesity Tight dressing Pneumo/hemothorax

FACTORS INFLUENCING ANALGESIC REQUIREMENT

1. Site

2. Sex : Female patients require opioids earlier, but total demand is equal.

3. Age : Elderly patients opioids requirements are low.

4. Personality :Analgesic requirements increased in patients with a neurotic personality.

5. Previous experience reduces demand, especially if the same operation is undertaken.

6. Response of patient : Huge variation in response to a given dose of drug- especially marked with opioids.

7. Motivation : Analgesia achieved more easily after surgery for benign conditions than after palliative cancer surgery.

MEDICAL GAS CYLINDERS

	Colour		Pressure at 15*C	
	Body	*Shoulder*	*lb f/in2*	*bar*
Oxygen	Black	White	1987	137
Nitrous oxide	Blue	Blue	638	44
Cyclopropane	Orange	Orange	73	5
CO_2	Grey	Grey	725	50
Helium	Brown	Brown	1987	137
Air	Grey	White/black quarters	1987	137
O_2/Helium	Black	White/brown quarters	1987	137
O_2/CO_2	Black	White/grey quarters	1987	137
N_2O/O_2 (Entonox)	Blue	White/blue quarters	1987	137

DOSES OF VARIOUS DRUGS USED FOR

A.	Premedication	Dose/Conc.
	Thiopentone (2.5% solution)	3-5 mg/kg
	Ketamine	1-2 mg/kg (I/V); 4-6 mg/kg (I/M)
	Curare	0.2-0.6 mg/kg
	Gallamine	1 mg/kg
	Pancuronium	0.04-0.12 mg/kg
	Scoline	1-1.5 mg/kg
	Morphine	0.15 mg/kg
	Pethidine	1.5 mg/kg
	Pentazocine	1-2 mg/kg
	Atropine (vagolytic)	0.01-0.02 mg/kg (Anti-Sialogogue) 0.02-0.04 mg/kg
	Dopamine	2.5 µg/kg/mt (upto 10)
	Lignocaine	1-2 mg/kg
B.	In cardiac arrest	
	Epinephrine	0.5-1.0 mg/kg I/V or Intracardiac (1 in 10,000)
	Sodium bicarbonate	1-2 meq/kg
	Calcium Chloride	5-10 CC of 10%
	KCI	5 c.c. of 4%

CIRCUITS USED FOR ANAESTHESIA

Mapelson A circuit	Heidbrink valve, Reservoir bag
Mepelson E system	Ayre's T-tube (used in Pediatrics)
Mepelson A system	Lack circuit
Mepelson D system	Bain circuit

IMPORTANT ADVERSE EFFECTS OF HIGH INSPIRED PRESSURES OF OXYGEN

Cardiovascular effects

Myocardial depression and vascular constriction. These effects are not clinically significant with 100% O_2 in healthy patients but may be overt in patients with severe cardiac disease.

Absorption atelectasis

Collapse of lung units may occur in 6 min with 100% O_2 60 min with 85% O_2 in the presence of airway closure.

CO_2 narcosis

Respiratory depression in patients with chronic chest disease and significant hypoxic ventilatory drive.

Pulmonary toxicity

Lung damage (capillary congestion, interstitial and alveolar oedema) is dependent on the partial pressure of oxygen and duration of exposure. Onset of oxygen-induced lung pathology occurs after approx. 30h exposure to PIO2 of 100 kPa.

CNS toxicity

Convulsions similar to grand mal epilepsy occur with exposure to hyperbaric pressures of O_2.

* **Effect of Anaesthesia on Respiratory Function**
  * FRC reduced
  * Change in breathing pattern with predominant diaphragmatic breathing (intercostals more depressed)
  * Reduced alveolar ventilation, depressed CO_2 response curve, reduced hypoxic respiratory drive
  * Increased shunt (increased (A-a) O_2 difference).
  * Increased dead space (physiological dead space).
  * Reduced compliance; increased resistance.
  * Increased V/Q abnormality (increased (A-a) O_2 difference).
  * Cilial paralysis, mucosal drying (anticholinergics, dry gas, nasal bypassing).
  * Airway instrumentation and contamination.
  * Depressed airway reflexes.

* **Positions for anaesthesia**

  Supine
  * Decreased FRC (about 30%) on assuming supine position. Further fall on induction of anaesthesia.
  * Restriction of diaphragmatic movement by abdominal contents (especially in obese patients).
  * Trachea angled backward (30°) in supine position so fluids will flow down.
  * Aortocaval compression (as described in pregnancy) can occur in the obese and in patients with intra-abdominal masses.
  * Flattening of the lumbar spine with muscle relaxation during anaesthesia, associated with flattening of the lumbar lordosis and post-operative backache.

  Trendelenburg
  * Further decrease of FRC over supine level.
  * Weight of abdominal contents splints diaphragm; increased work of breathing.
  * Increased venous return, increased cerebral venous pressure (reduced cerebral perfusion pressure, raised ICP).
  * Raised intragastric pressure.
  * Shoulder pressure can cause brachial plexus injury.

  Reverse Trendlenburg
  * Venous pooling and reduced venous return.
  * Lesser fall of FRC than in supine position.

Lithotomy

* Decreased vital capacity and FRC (restriction of diaphragm, especially in obese patients).
* Increased work of breathing.
* Increased intragastric pressure.
* Difficulty in turning patients in emergency (legs secured).
* Danger of injuries to hips and backs.
* Risk of pressure damage to common peroneal nerve if legs positioned inside poles.

Lateral

* Better ventilation in lower lung during spontaneous respiration (lower dome of diaphragm is raised by abdominal contents so greater potential for excursion, also more curved so more force - (application of Laplace's law), also more blood flow to lower long (gravity effect).
* Lack of stability (patient must by supported).
* Decreased ventilation of lower lung during IPPV leads to increased V/Q inequality.

Prone

* Reduced antero-posterior (A-P) chest expansion.
* Diaphragmatic excursion can be restricted when support of the shoulders and pelvis is incorrect (especially in obese patients).
* Eyes must be protected from abrasion.
* Difficulty in holding on mask and maintaining airway.
* Poor access to the endotracheal tube; possibility of tube kinking during positioning.
* Brachial plexus damage if arms brought too far forward.

MCQ's OF MISCELLANEOUS

What is important in Miscellaneous

Causes of difficult intubation, Common complications during anaesthesia (hypotension, arrythmias, pneumothorax, hypertension, vomiting, hypoventilation, intracranial pressure), Apparatus (Magill's circuits, Boyle's apparatus), I/V solutions, endotracheal tube size estimation, Important drug interactions, Anaesthesia in special situations (Children/Elderly/Pregnancy/Diabetes mellitus/Porphyria/Neuro or CVS surgery etc.), Important Physiological Factual data (Boiling temp. and partition coefficients of anaesthetics), Respiratory, Liver and Kidney function tests etc.

1. **Raised intracranial pressure in posterior cranial fossa cause all of the following except:**

   AIIMS 1984, 90
   A. Hypertension   B. Bradycardia
   C. Bradypnoea   D. Frontal headache

2. **Slow reacting substance of anaphylaxis is a mixture of the following Leukotriens except :**   **DNB 1993**
   A. LTB_4 B. LTC_4
   C. LTD_4 D. LTE_4

3. **The value of minimal alveolar concentration is not altered by:**   **DNB 1988**
   A. Age   B. Narcotics
   C. Guanethidine   D. Alpha-methyldopa
   E. Body temperature

4. **When wheezing occurs intraoperatively, appropriate measure may include all of the following except:**

   AIIMS 1982
   A. The intratracheal administration of mucolytic agents.
   B. Use of a volatile anaesthetic agent (e.g. halothane)
   C. Rechecking breath sound bilaterally.
   D. Intravenous hydrocortisone.
   E. Determination of arterial PO_2, PCO_2, and pH.

5. **Cerebral metabolic rate and cerebral blood flow are not reduced by:**   **Delhi 1987**
   A. Ketamine   B. Morphine
   C. Thiopental   D. Diazepam
   E Halothane

6. **Cholinesterase metabolises the following except :**

   PGI 1997
   A. Propanidid   B. Procaine
   C. Acetylcholine   D. Scoline

7. **Bain system is modification of:**   **Delhi 1985**
   A. Mepelson A system   B. Mapelson B system
   C. Mapelson C system   D. Mapelson D system

8. **At a flow rate of 3L/min, inspiratory O_2 (FI02) concentration of 24% can be achieved by using a :**

   UPSC 1997
   A. Nasopharyngeal catheter
   B. Simple face mask
   C. Venturi mask
   D. Head box

9. **The treatment and prevention of disease and the management of pain by puncturing the skin needles is termed as :**   **AMU 1986**
   A. Conduction Anaesthesia
   B. Refrigeration analgesia
   C. Field block
   D. Acupunture
   E. Neurolept Analgesia

10. **Hyperbaric oxygen has----- atmospheric pressure.**

    Delhi 1996
    A. 0.3   B. 0.5
    C. 1   D. 2

11. **The thoracic index is :**   **DNB 1990**
    A. The ratio between coronal and longitudinal diameters of the thorax.
    B. The ratio between sagittal and transverse diameters of the thorax.
    C. Highest in the fetus.
    D. Only A and B are true.
    E. Only B and C are true.

Ans.   1. D   2. A   3. C   4. A   5. A   6. A   7. D   8. C   9. D   10. D
11. E

12. Choose the incorrect statement :   AIIMS 1986
    A. In steal syndrome hypercarbia causes vasodilation in normal cerebral vessels and divert blood from disease to healthy areas.
    B. In Luxary perfusion there is a localized over abundant cerebral blood flow relative to metabolic need and is commonly seen around area of damaged brain.
    C. Heat causes cerebral vasoconstriction while cold has the reverse effect.
    D. Total cerebral blood flow in a normal adult is approximately 750 ml/minute.
    E. The critical value for cerebral blood flow rate is about 30 ml/100g/minute of brain.

13. The classical position commonly used in Neurosurgery includes all of the following except :   AIIMS 1986
    A. Supine   B. Prone
    C. Sitting   D. Standing
    E. Lateral

14. Risk of air embolism occur in which of the following positions, during neurosurgical operation :   AIIMS 1986
    A. Supine   B. Prone
    C. Sitting   D. Lateral

15. APGAR score is used to evaluate :   DNB 1990
    A. Cerebral anoxia   B. Maternal mortality
    C. Foetal asphyxia   D. Cardiac risk

16. The prediction of correct endotracheal tube size is probably most accurately based upon the child's :   Rohtak 1986
    A. Length   B. Age
    C. Body weight   D. Body surface area
    E. None of the above

17. The important source of energy in the neonate which also maintains the body heat is :   DNB 1991
    A. Muscle   B. Liver
    C. Brown Fat   D. Myocardium
    E. Breakdown of R.B.C.

18. Neonate Emergencies requiring surgery immediately include all of the following except :   AMU 1986
    A. Diaphragmatic Hernia
    B. Cleft Palate
    C. Tracheo-Oesophageal Fistula
    D. Neonatal intestinal obstruction
    E. Mandibular Retrognathia

19. Resuscitation bag volume in neonates should not exceed :   JIPMER 1998
    A. 240 ml   B. 500 ml
    C. 750 ml   D. 1000 ml

20. In managing severe respiratory depression of the new-born all efforts should be made to correct :   AIIMS 1982
    A. Hypoventilation   B. Hypoxia
    C. Hypercarbia   D. All of the above
    E. Only B and C are true

21. Breathing 100% oxygen, pulmonary oxygen toxicity does not occur in an environment of :   BHU 1986
    A. 0.5 ATA   B. 1.0 ATA
    C. 1.5 ATA   D. 2.0 ATA
    E. 3.0 ATA

22. The vasodilator effect of isoproternol can be abolished by :   AMU 1986
    A. Chlorpromazine   B. Hydralazine
    C. Phenoxybenzamine   D. Propranolol
    E. Trimethaphan

23. Stellate ganglion is formed by the fusion of the :   PGI 1985
    A. Lowest of the three cervical ganglion with the first thoracic ganglion.
    B. Superior and middle cervical ganglion.
    C. Middle and inferior cervical ganglion.
    D. Superior, middle and inferior cervical ganglion.
    E. None of the above.

24. Prominent tubercle palpable behind the lateral border of sternomastoid muscle is of the :   AMU 1985
    A. Fifth cervical vertebra
    B. Sixth cervical vertebra
    C. Seventh cervical vertebra
    D. First thoracic vertebra
    E. None of the above

25. Felypressin is a :   PGI 1982
    A. Vasoconstrictor
    B. Vasodilator
    C. Anticholinesterase
    D. Para-sympatholytic agent
    E. Ganglion stimulating agent

26. Commonest complication of I.V. infusion in comatose child is :   JIPMER 1993
    A. Overdehydration   B. Hyponatremia
    C. Hyperkalemia   D. Hypothermia

Ans.	12. C	13. D	14. C	15. C	16. B	17. C	18. B	19. A	20. D	21. A
	22. D	23. A	24. B	25. A	26. D					

27. Composition of sodalime is :   Delhi 1993, 96

	Na OH	Ca (OH)$_2$	KOH
A.	4%	95%	1%
B.	20%	80%	—
C.	80%	20%	—
D.	15%	84%	1%

28. Stellate ganglion block is characterized by following except :   Delhi 1993
    A. Miosis   B. Ptosis
    C. Flushing   D. Sweating

29. Multisystem injury with - CVP with fluctuating BP is: Delhi 1992
    A. Subdural hematoma
    B. Unrecognised chest injury
    C. Abdominal bleeding
    D. Airway obstruction

30. Which of the following agents crosses the placenta the quickest :   Delhi 1993
    A. Thiopentone   B. Morphine
    C. Gallamine   D. d-TC

31. Part of which a cylinder containing anaesfilling gases is attached is termed as :   PGI 1983
    A. Cylinder outlet valve   B. Pin Index
    C. Yokes   D. Reducing valve
    E. Venturi

32. Non-Rebreathing valves have all the following advantage except :   AIIMS 1982
    A. Wastage of expensive agent and atmospheric pollution.
    B. Can be used for spontaneous or controlled respiration.
    C. Can measure Minute Volume if flowmetres are accurate.
    D. No possibility of CO_2 build-up if valve dead space is small.

33. On arrival in the recovery room, the patient is not responding and pale but is breathing well and is normotensive. The PAR score on the Aldrete scale is: AIIMS 1982
    A. 3   B. 4
    C. 5   D. 6
    E. 7

34. It is characteristic of high-frequency osscillatory ventilation that :   AIIMS 1982
    A. It is very similar to high-frequency positive pressure ventilation.
    B. It accomplishes gas exchange without bulk air exchange.
    C. It is used at the rate of 300 to 500 strokes/min.
    D. There is an appreciable net flow of gas in the trachea.
    E. Pulmonary overdistention is a very real risk.

35. Biochemical changes occurring during Hypercapnia includes all of the following except :   AIIMS 1984
    A. pH changes i.e. Respiratory acidosis
    B. Compensatory metabolic alkalosis, Secretion of acid urine with retention of bicarbonate and sodium.
    C. Rise in Serum Potassium.
    D. Rise of plasma 15-Hydroxycorticosteroids.
    E. None of the above.

36. The most sensitive diagnostic method for recognizing venous air embolism is :   AIIMS 1986
    A. End tidal CO_2
    B. Direct arterial pressure
    C. Central venous pressure
    D. Alterations in respiratory patterns
    E. Precordial Doppler monitoring

37. In the management of a patient with severe aortic stenosis it is important to maintain :   AIIMS 1986
    A. Maximum beta-blockage
    B. Low arterial impedance to blood flow
    C. Properly timed atrial contractions
    D. Sinus tachycardia
    E. A low preload

38. The anaesthetic managment of the patients with IHSS should include all of the following except :   AIIMS 1984
    A. Halothane as the principle anaesthetic agent.
    B. The maintenance of a high preload.
    C. Use of the pure alpha-adrenergic agonists if vasopressors are indicated.
    D. The avoidance or immediate treatment of tachycardia.

39. The human blood product with the lowest risk of hepatitis transmission is :   AIIMS 1983
    A. Whole blood
    B. Salt-poor albumin
    C. Fresh-frozen plasma
    D. Frozen washed red blood cells
    E. Factor concentrates

40. Dangers, commonly associated with the upright position in neurosurgical position include/s :   AIIMS 1984
    A. Air Embolism   B. Severe Hypotension
    C. Both of the above   D. None of the above

41. The most effective positions undoubtedly, for producing an uncongesting field for a cervical laminectomy or posterior fossa craniotomy is :   AIIMS 1985
    A. Sitting   B. Supine
    C. Lateral   D. Prone
    E. None of the above

Ans.	27. A	28. D	29. B	30. A	31. C	32. A	33. C	34. B	35. E	36. E
	37. C	38. D	39. B	40. C	41. A					

42. **The basis of good anaesthesia for neurosurgery is/ are :**   **AIIMS 1985**
    A. Perfect airway for Adequate Ventilation.
    B. Low venous pressure and a slack brain.
    C. Minimal bleeding and absence of coughing or straining.
    D. Rapid return to consciousness.
    E. All of the above.

43. **Armoured Endotracheal tubes, whose walls are reinforced with a nylon spiral, are good for :**   **AIIMS 1980**
    A. Peadiatric Anaesthesia
    B. Cardio vascular surgery Anaesthesia
    C. Neuro Surgical Anaesthesia
    D. Obstetric Anaesthesia
    E. Respiratory Anaesthesia

44. **Remedial measures for reduction of Intracranial tension during Neuro surgical anaesthesia, both Pre-operative and perioperative include :**   **BHU 1985**
    A. Hyperventilation with use of muscle relaxants
    B. Use of hyperosmotic agents
    C. Induced hypotension
    D. Use of steroids
    E. All of the above

45. **Clinical signs of venous air embolism include all of the following except :**   **DNB 1991**
    A. Cardiac arrythmias
    B. Rising end expiratory CO_2
    C. Neck vein distention
    D. Changes in the heart beat
    E. Bronchospasm

46. **The characteristic feature(s) of a competitive block is (are):**   **AMU 1987**
    A. T sustained contraction produced by tetanic stimulation.
    B. The possibility of a dual block.
    C. The potentiation by neostigmine.
    D. The presence of post-tetanic facilitation.

47. **Which of the following suppresses ADH release:**   **AMU 1987**
    A. Morphine
    B. Angiotensin
    C. Intracranial hypertension
    D. Atropine
    E. Thiopental

48. **Why the SA node normally is the pacemaker of the heart:**   **CMC 1987**
    A. Because of its location in the atrium.
    B. Because of its strength of the impulse formation.
    C. Because of its rate of impulse formation.
    D. Because of neural control.
    E. Because of its proximity to the AV node.

49. **Para sympathetic stimulation of the heart results in:**   **AMU 1986**
    A. An increase in the AV junctional fibres.
    B. A decrease in the rate of discharge of the AV node.
    C. A prevention of ventricular contractions.
    D. A decreased permeability to nodal cells of K^+.
    E. A decrease in conduction velocity.

50. **Optical oxygen transport occurs when the hematocrit is:**   **BHU 1986**
    A. Between 30% and 35%
    B. Between 40% and 45%
    C. Between 46% and 54%
    D. Between 55% and 65%
    E. Optical oxygen transport is independent of the hematocrit.

51. **In which part of the cardiovascular system is the largest volume of blood located:**   **DNB 1989**
    A. The heart   B. The large arteries
    C. The capillaries   D. The large veins
    D. The pulmonary artery

52. **Which part of the circulatory system has the largest total cross-section area :**   **Delhi 1990**
    A. The large arteries   B. The arteries
    C. The capillaries   D. The small veins
    E. The large veins

53. **Brainstem auditory-evoked potentials cannot be used to :**   **PGI 1987**
    A. Test hearing in infants.
    B. Assess brainstem function in comatose.
    C. Monitor the eighth cranial nerve during surgical procedures.
    D. Monitor the brainstem during posterior cranial fossa exploration.
    E. Monitor ascending spinal tracts during scoliosis surgery.

54. **The greatest drop in systemic arterial blood pressure occurs in——— vessels.**   **PGI 1984**
    A. Capacitance
    B. Venules
    C. Pre-capillary resistance
    D. None of the above

Ans.	42. E	43. C	44. E	45. B	46. D	47. D	48. C	49. B	50. B	51. D
	52. C	53. E	54. C							

55. In mitral stenosis, an established case, the area of (sq.cm.) of mitral office is reduced to :   DNB 1990
A. 5.5   B. 4.5
C. 3.5   D. 2.5
E. 1.5

56. Propranolol is indicated in :   PGI 1982
A. High Renin Hypertension
B. Low Renin Hypertension
C. Normal Renin Hypertension
D. All of the above
E. None of the above

57. E.C.G. changes in digitalis toxicity includes all of the following except :   DNB 1990
A. Complete heart block
B. Sinus Tachycardia
C. ST segment depression
D. Ventricular extrasystole
E. None of the following

58. In Anaesthetic pratice, pre-operative digitalization may be considered in order to prevent :   DNB 1991
A. Intra-cardiac failure
B. Supra-ventricular dysrhythmias.
C. Post-operative cardiac failure
D. All of the obove
E. Only A and B are true.

59. During anaesthesia, digoxin toxicity may be precipitated by: AIIMS 1982
A. Changes in catecholamine levels
B. Changes in Pottasium or sodium level
C. By use of drugs such as Suxamethonium
D. Alteration in pH consequent on changes in ventilation
E. All of the obove

60. Somatosensory-evoked potential monitoring may be most helpful in which operation :   AIIMS 1983
A. Posterior fossa exploration
B. Carotid endarterectomy
C. Resection of pituitary tumours
D. Middle ear surgery in infants
E. Thoracic aorta surgery

61. Circulation can be arrested safely for 30 minutes at a core temperature of :   AIIMS 1985
A. 5° to 10°   B. 10° to 15°
C. 15° to 20°   D. 20° to 30°
E. 25° to 30°

62. During deep hypothermia, the brain temperature is measured most accurately in the :   Rohtak 1987
A. Skin

B. Esophagus
C. Rectum
D. Middle ear (tympanic membrane)
E. Nasopharynx

63. Emergence delirium is most commonly associated with :   Delhi 1989
A. Phenothiazines
B. Diazepam
C. Tricyclic antidepressants
D. Belladonna alkaloids
E. Antiparkinsonian drugs

64. Cauda Equina syndrome is neurological sequelae which may occur after :   PGI 1982
A. General anaesthesia   B. Spinal anaesthesia
C. Epidural anaesthesia   D. None of the above

65. Dopamine is :   AI 1986
A. An alpha agonist
B. Primarily a beta agonist
C. An alpha blocking agent
D. A beta blocking agent

66. What is the reasonable size for an endotracheal tube to be used in an average 3-years old child :   AIIMS 1986
A. 2 mm   B. 4.5 mm
C. 5.5 mm   D. 6 mm

67. Raised pCO_2 indicates :   AIIMS 1986
A. Bronchial asthma
B. Pulmonary fibrosis
C. Alveolar hyperventilation
D. Alveolar hypoventilation

68. Optimal decrease in ICP can be achieved at a $PaCO_2$ of :   AMU 1987
A. 35 mm Hg   B. 30 mm Hg
C. 25 mm Hg   D. 20 mm Hg
E. Below 20 mm Hg

69. The basic rational for IMV is that :   AIIMS 1982
A. It is less expensive.
B. There are varying degrees of acute and chronic respiratory insufficiencies.
C. It requires less sophisticated equipment.
D. It requires minimal monitoring.
E. It completely protects the apnoeic patient.

70. With an FIO2 of 1 at 3 ATA, the amount of oxygen dissolved in the plasma will be :   AIIMS 1984
A. 0.3 mL   B. 0.6 mL
C. 2.0 mL   D. 4.0 mL
E. 6.0 mL

Ans.	55. D	56. A	57. B	58. D	59. E	60. E	61. B	62. D	63. D	64. B
	65. B	66. B	67. D	68. B	69. B	70. E				

71. **The simplest method of decreasing intracranial pressure is to :**   **DNB 1990**
    A. Intubate and hyperventilate the patient.
    B. Do a lumbar puncture and drain off CSF.
    C. Induce diuresis.
    D. Elevate the head of the bed by 30°.
    E. Use acetazolamide.

72. **If a patient has a chronic respiratory acidosis and the $PaCO_2$ is 60 mm Hg, the predicated pH will be :**   **Delhi 1982**
    A. 7.20   B. 7.25
    C. 7.30   D. 7.36
    E. 7.40

73. **When a patient is breathing air at 3 ATA, the end tidal CO_2 tension will be approximately :**   **Delhi 1982**
    A. 40 mm Hg   B. 80 mm Hg
    C. 120 mm Hg   D. 240 mm Hg
    E. 760 mm Hg

74. **Change in Respiratory Acidosis that occurs in blood include :**   **UPSC 1988**
    A. pCO_2 rises, Plasma bicarbonate rises, pH falls.
    B. pCO_2 rises, Plasma bicarbonate falls, pH rises.
    C. pCO_2 falls, Plasma bicarbonate rises, pH falls.
    D. pCO_2 falls, Plasma bicarbonate falls, pH falls.

75. **Respiratory Alkalosis commonly occurs during :**   **Delhi 1984**
    A. Diabetic Coma
    B. Spontaneous Ventilation
    C. Controlled Ventilation
    D. Badly choosen or malfunctioning apparatus
    E. Severe Pyloric stenosis

76. **Metabolic acidosis may occur in all of the following conditions except :**   **BHU 1987**
    A. Diabetic Ketosis and starvation
    B. Associated with "Neostigmine resistant curarization".
    C. Following cardiac arrest.
    D. During cardio-pulmonary bypass causing hypoxia.
    E. Severe Pyloric stenosis.

77. **Causes of Hypercapnia in anaesthetic practice includes all of the following except :**   **Delhi 1989**
    A. Gross impairment of ventilation due to respiratory obstruction, profound narcosis or relaxant.
    B. Accidental administration of CO_2.
    C. During controlled respiration.
    D. Faulty CO_2 absorption, e.g worn out soda lime in circuit.
    E. The technique of apnoeic insufflation oxygenation.

78. **Effects of hypercapnia on central nervous system are :**   **Bihar 1990**
    A. Increased cerebral blood flow, and CSF pressure.
    B. Impairment of mental activity and loss of consciousness.
    C. Stimulation of Respiration initially.
    D. Progressive Narcosis.
    E. All of the above.

79. **The only indication/s of Hypercapnia during anaesthesia is/are :**   **AMU 1987**
    A. Increase in depth of respiration
    B. Difficulty in controlling the ventilation
    C. Blood pressure falls
    D. Both A and B are true

80. **All the following cause bronchodilation except :**   **JIPMER 1992**
    A. Salbutamol   B. Thiopentone
    C. Ether   D. Neostigmine

81. **Treatment of Intracranial tension is following except :**   **JIPMER 1992**
    A. I.V. Frusemide
    B. I.V. Mannitol
    C. Controlled hyperventilation
    D. Positive end pressure ventilation

82. **All of the following decrease CO2 absorption in circuit except :**   **AIIMS 1992**
    A. ↑ resistance in circuit   B. ↑ flow
    C. ↓ dead space   D. ↑ tidal volume

83. **All of the following cause late respiratory depression except :**   **PGI 1993**
    A. Morphine   B. Buprenorphine
    C. Fentanyl   D. Pethidine

84. **The rate flow of fresh gases through Ayre's T-tube in 1 year old is :**   **PGI 1993**
    A. 3-4 L/mm   B. 5-6 L/mm
    C. 6-7 L/mm   D. 8-9 L/mm

85. **Mendelson syndrome occurs due to :**   **JIPMER 1993**
    A. Aspiration of gastric contents
    B. Nitrous Oxide overdosage
    C. Acidosis
    D. High pressure airleak

86. **In doing a phrenic nerve block, it is best to infiltrate:**   **AIIMS 1986**
    A. Scalenus anterior
    B. Scalenus posterior
    C. Posterior border of sternomastoid
    D. Anterior border of sternomastoid

Ans.	71. D	72. D	73. A	74. A	75. C	76. E	77. C	78. E	79. D	80. B
	81. D	82. A	83. B	84. C	85. A	86. A				

87. The most valuable indication of anaesthetic over-dose is : **AIIMS 1985**

A. Tachycardia   B. Hypotension
C. Cardiac arrhythmias   D. Depressed respiration
E. Pupillary size

88. Sodium hydroxide in soda lime acts as : **AIIMS 1981**

A. A catalyst   B. A humdifying agent
C. An indicator   D. All of the above

89. Muscarinic effects of acetylcholine occur on all of the following except : **Delhi 1982**

A. Secretory glands   B. Myocardium
C. Pupil   D. Skeletal muscle

90. Acquired methaemoglobinaemia, caused by a number of drugs and chemical includes all except : **AMU 1987**

A. Nitrates   B. Phenacetin
C. Prilocaine   D. Sulphanilamide
E. None of the above

91. Methaemoglobinaemia differs from sulphaemoglobinaemia in that the former : **PGI 1986**

A. Gives a chocolate brown appearance
B. Wave of their absorption spectra is unequal
C. It can be treated
D. All of the above
E. None of the above

92. The acquired from of methaemoglobinaemia can be treated by all of the following except : **PGI 1986**

A. Removal of causative agent
B. I.V. 1% of Methylene blue (1-2 mg/kg body weight)
C. Vit. C 500 mg/diem
D. Oral methylene blue
E. Both C and D are true

93. Inotropic agent of choice in a child with pulmonary arterial hypertension is : **DNB 1990**

A. Dobutamine   B. Isoprenaline
C. Dopamine   D. Afrenaline

94. The goals of management in the post-operative period in a child who has undergone Fontan procedure include all of the following except : **AIIMS 1983**

A. Maintenance of CVP at a higher level (15-20 cm of H_2O)
B. Early extubation
C. Overnight mechanical ventilation
D. Tachycardia

95. One of the following represents cyanotic heart disease with increased pulmonary blood flow : **DNB 1989**

A. Transposition of the great arteries
B. Ebstein's anamoly
C. Tetralogy of Fallot
D. VSD with reversal of shunt

96. Post-operative complications following surgery for the correction of coarctation of descending aorta include all of the following except : **AIIMS 1983**

A. Hypertension   B. Paraplegia
C. Bowel ischaemia   D. Hypothermia

97. The normal systolic and diastolic pressure respectively in a normal right ventricle are : **AIIMS 1983**

A. 25/8 mm Hg   B. 45/10 mm Hg
C. 50/25 mm Hg   D. 60/20 mm Hg

98. Recommended respiratory management after VSD repair in a patient with pulmonary hypertension is : **DNB 1986**

A. Elective mechanical ventilation and extubation within 6 to 8 hours.
B. Extubation on the table and oxygen administration by polymask in the ICU.
C. Elective overnight mechanical ventilation.
D. Continuous positive airway pressure (CPAP).

99. A common type of dysrhythmia associated with WPW syndrome is : **Delhi 1983**

A. Atrial flutter
B. Ventricular tachycardia
C. Paraoxysmal supra-ventricular tachycardia
D. Atrial fibrillation

100. One of the following is an ultra short-acting beta adrenergic blocker : **DNB 1991**

A. Timolol   B. Esmolol
C. Pindolol   D. Nadolol

101. In a child who has undergone a left sided BT shunt for TOF : **AIIMS 1985**

A. The right radial artery pulsations are absent.
B. The left radial artery pulsations are absent.
C. The right femoral artery pulsations are absent.
D. The left radial artery pulsations are bounding.

102. Uterine blood flow is not reduced by : **AP 1991**

A. Ephedrine
B. Positive-pressure ventilation
C. Maternal hypotension
D. Methoxamine
E. Epinephrine

Ans.	87. B	88. A	89. D	90. E	91. D	92. E	93. B	94. C	95. A	96. D
	97. A	98. C	99. C	100. B	101. B	102. A				

103. The anticholinesterase agents :   **Bihar 1990**
   A. Relax the ureteric and bronchiolar smooth muscles.
   B. Decreases the resting rate of secretion in the exocrine glands.
   C. Produce anhydrosis.
   D. Cause bradycardia and a decrease in cardiac output.
   E. Decrease the acidity of gastric secretions.

104. Which of the following prevents the release of cholinergic transmitter :   **DNB 1991**
   A. Bretylium   B. Iproniazid
   C. Botulinum toxin   D. Nicotine
   E. Neostigmine

105. Verapamil must be used very carefully in the presence of :   **Delhi 1987**
   A. Amnioglycosides
   B. High cervical spinal injury
   C. Extensive burns
   D. Tricyclic antidepressants
   E. Beta-adrenergic blocking agents

106. Pupillary constriction caused by morphine is :   **AMU 1986**
   A. Due to local action on the pupillary sphincter muscle.
   B. No longer evident as tolerance develops.
   C. Accompanied by increased intraocular pressure.
   D. Due to stimulation of the Edinger Westphal nucleus.
   E. Due to action on medullary centres.

107. After massive transfusion the most important blood component to administer is :   **AIIMS 1986**
   A. Platelets   B. Cryoprecipitate
   C. Fibrinogen   D. Fresh-frozen plasma
   E. Washed red cells

108. The dose of bicarbonate to correct a base deficit of 10 mEq/L in a 155-lb male is approximately :   **AIIMS 1982**
   A. 44 mEq   B. 60 mEq
   C. 106 mEq   D. 155 mEq
   E. 233 mEq

109. Which of the following circulatory parameters is not increased during closed-chest cardiac compression :   **AMU 1986**
   A. Aortic pressure
   B. Jugular vein pressure
   C. Systolic arterial pressure
   D. Coronary blood flow
   E. Carotid blood flow

110. Levodopa should be discontinued how may hours prior to anaesthesia :   **DNB 1991**
   A. 4 hours   B. 12 hours
   C. 24 hours   D. 48 hours

111. In the treatment of persistent ventricular arrhythmias, the recommended infusion rate of lidocaine is ———mg/kg/min.   **AIIMS 1986**
   A. 5.0 to 10.0   B. 2.0 to 4.0
   C. 1.0 to 1.5   D. 0.5 to 1.0
   E. 0.1 to 0.5

112. If a vasopressor is to be used in haemorrhagic shock, the best drug is :   **DNB 1991**
   A. Norepinephrine   B. Epinephrine
   C. Dobutamine   D. Dopamine
   E. Phenylephrine

113. In severe polycythemia, the viscosity of the blood may be :   **DNB 1989**
   A. The same as water
   B. Twice the viscosity of water
   C. 5 times the viscosity of water
   D. 10 times the viscosity of water
   E. 25 times the viscosity of water

114. Drugs that improve cardiac contractility includes all except :   **AIIMS 1982**
   A. Calcium   B. Glucagon
   C. Dipamine   D. Aminophylline
   E. Digoxin

115. The normal blood volume for an adult may be taken as ——— percent of body weight.   **Delhi 1988**
   A. 6.7   B. 7.7
   C. 8.7   D. 9.7
   E. 10.7

116. Conditions or drugs which causes rise of CVP include all except :   **PGI 1984**
   A. I.P.P.V   B. Heart failure
   C. Nitroprusside   D. Valsalava manoeuvre
   E. Catecholamines

117. Conditions and/or drug which causes lowering of CVP include all except :   **AIIMS 1985**
   A. Hypovolaemia
   B. Ganglion Blockers
   C. Vomiting
   D. Standing upright
   E. Reduction of venous tone by unconsciousness

118. Which is a more dangerous condition :   **DNB 1990**
   A. Partial block   B. Unstable block
   C. Stable complete block D. Both A and B are true
   E. Both A and C are true

Ans.	103. D	104. C	105. E	106. D	107. A	108. E	109. B	110. A	111. C	112. D
	113. B	114. C	115. B	116. C	117. C	118. D				

119. A History of Stokes-Adams attacks, giddiness, collapse or fainting suggests :   **AIIMS 1982**
   A. Complete block   B. Unstable block
   C. Hemi block   D. All of the above
   E. Only A and C are true

120. Chassignae's tubercle is :   **AIIMS 1984**
   A. Below the level of cricoid cartilage
   B. Above the level of cricoid cartilage
   C. At the same level as cricoid cartilage
   D. Present at C7 level

121. For brachial plexus block, needle is inserted :   **AIIMS 1986**
   A. Medial to subclavian artery
   B. Lateral to subclavian artery
   C. Medial to subclavian artery
   D. Lateral to subclavian artery

122. Carina in an adult is at the level of :   **Rohtak 1987**
   A. T2   B. T3
   C. T4   D. T6

123. Gag reflex can be depressed by blocking one of the following cranial nerves :   **Rohtak 1987**
   A. V   B. IX
   C. X   D. XII

124. An adult trachea has a diameter of :   **DNB 1989**
   A. 0.5-1 cm   B. 1.2-1.6 cms
   C. 2.5-3 cms   D. 3-3.5 cms

125. The length of an adult trachea is :   **DNB 1983**
   A. 6 to 8 cm   B. 10 to 11 cm
   C. 14 to 15 cm   D. 16 to 20 cm

126. In an adult, right bronchus is angled from the vertical at :   **PGI 1984**
   A. 10°   B. 25°
   C. 45°   D. 55°

127. In a neonate, both bronchi are angled from the vertical at :   **AIIMS 1985**
   A. 10°   B. 25°
   C. 45°   D. 55°

128. During deep breathing contribution of the diaphragm to tidal volume is :   **AIIMS 1984**
   A. 30%   B. 50%
   C. 85%   D. 100%

129. If the cardiac output is doubled in a normal human, the mean pulmonary artery pressure will :   **AIIMS 1983**
   A. Remain normal or increase slightly
   B. Double
   C. Quadruple
   D. Decrease by 50%
   E. Decrease by 25%

130. What is the proportion between left ventricular stroke-work output and right ventricular stroke-work output :   **AIIMS 1983**
   A. 1 : 1   B. 2 : 1
   C. 7 : 1   D. 15 : 1
   E. 22 : 1

131. The largest drop in pressure occurs in which part of the vascular system :   **Delhi 1982**
   A. The arteries   B. The arterioles
   C. The capillaries   D. The small veins
   E. The large veins

132. What happens when the CSF pressure approaches the level of arterial pressure :   **AIIMS 1986**
   A. The arterial pressure falls.
   B. The cerebrovascular resistence decreases.
   C. The flow of CSF is reversed.
   D. The Cushing reflex raises arterial pressure.
   E. There will be no change in the sytemic circulation

133. In normal humans, coronary artery blood flow is primarily controlled by :   **AMU 1986**
   A. Sympathetic impulses
   B. Parasympathetic impulse
   C. Hypocardia
   D. Myocardial O_2 demand
   E. Hypercardia

134. The alpha receptors for adrenergic impulses are found in :   **AP 1991**
   A. The SA node
   B. The atria of the heart
   C. The ventricles of the heart
   D. The bronchial muscles
   E. The salivary glands

135. All of the following are effects of smoking except :   **Delhi 1984**
   A. Increase in mathaemoglobin
   B. Vasoconstriction
   C. Decreased mucociliary action
   D. Increased closing volume

136. One of the following chemotherapeutic drug causes inhibition of pseudocholinesterase :   **Delhi 1984**
   A. Vinblastine   B. Methotrexate
   C. Cyclophosphamide   D. Vincristine

137. All the following drugs act at the dopaminergic receptors except :   **AIIMS 1984**
   A. Haloperidol   B. Domperidone
   C. Metoclopramide   D. Dobutamine

Ans.	119. A	120. C	121. B	122. C	123. B	124. B	125. B	126. B	127. D	128. C
	129. A	130. C	131. B	132. D	133. D	134. E	135. A	136. C	137. D	

138. Thermoregulation mechanism is present in all vaporizers except : **PGI 1983**
    A. E.M.O.   B. Drager
    C. Copper kettle   D. Ohio

139. After the rapid infusion of 250 ml whole blood, the blood pressure falls and there is marked oozing at the operative site. The most likely diagnosis is : **DNB 1986**
    A. An allergic reaction   B. A hemolytic reaction
    C. Citrate intoxication   D. Circulatory overload
    E. Hypothermia

140. The most common coagulopathy following massive transfusion is due to : **BHU 1988**
    A. DIC
    B. Citrate intoxication
    C. Metabolic acidosis
    D. Dilutional coagulopathy
    E. Hemolytic reaction

141. In a previously healthy adult acute blood loss is considered significant if it exceeds : **AMU 1985**
    A. 2% of blood volume   B. 5% of blood volume
    C. 10% of blood volume   D. 15% of blood volume
    E. 20% of blood volume

142. In stored blood, there is an excess of following except : **Delhi 1982**
    A. Ammonia   B. Hydrogen ions
    C. Plasma potassium D. 2, 3 DPG

143. The treatment of choice in hypofibrinogenemia may include the administration of following except : **Delhi 1982**
    A. Heparin   B. Fresh plasma
    C. EACA   D. Dextran

144. Best preservative for blood : **WB 1998**
    A. ACD   B. CPD
    C. Heparin   D. EDTA

145. Pulse oximetry is based on : **WB 1998**
    A. Leplace's law   B. Boyles law
    C. Beer-lambert's law   D. Rammon effect

146. Intubation granuloma occurs in : **WB 1998**
    A. Ant. Commissure
    B. Junction of Ant. 1/3 & Post. 1/3rd
    C. Posterior 1/3rd
    D. Supra glottic

147. In an unconscious patient, ventilation is best maintained by : **WB 1998**
    A. Tracheostomy
    B. Cuffed endotracheal tube
    C. Non-cuffed endotracheal
    D. Oral intubation

148. In an elderly patient who presents for anorectal surgery which position during anaesthesia is likely to complicate apnoea : **Bihar 1998**
    A. Trendlenburg's   B. Reverse Trendlenburgs
    C. Supine   D. Prone

149. Highly lipid soluble agent would be associated with: **MAHE 1998**
    A. Potent anaesthesia action
    B. Potent analgesic action
    C. Excellent muscle relaxant action
    D. Least respiratory depression

150. Fasciculation is not expected as a result of : **Delhi 1982**
    A. Calcium deficiency
    B. Benign myokymia
    C. Injection of gallamine
    D. Injection of decamethonium
    E. Herniated nucleus pulposus

151. Oxygen concentration in mixed venous blood is ------ mm Hg. **Delhi 1996**
    A. 40   B. 60
    C. 70   D. 80

152. Consciousness is lost when one breathes air at a height from sea level of : **PGI 1982**
    A. 19,000 feet   B. 21,000 feet
    C. 23,000 feet   D. 33,000 feet
    E. 35,000 feet

153. The Heidbrink Meter in Boyle Machine : **AP 1990**
    A. Reduces pressure of gases
    B. Indicate flow rate of gases
    C. Humidity the anaesthetic gases
    D. Is a fixed orifice meter
    E. Is a Vaporizer

154. Gastric emptying time is increased when standard doses of the following are given except : **DNB 1990**
    A. Aspirin   B. Scopolamine
    C. Morphine D. Methadone

155. Non-inhalation gas that can be used for sterilization : **DNB 1990**
    A. Nitrogen   B. Xenon
    C. Helium   D. Ethylene oxide
    E. Ethylene

156. Low serum cholinesterase levels are seen in all of the following conditions except : **Delhi 1984**
    A. Cardiac failure   B. Hyperpyrexia
    C. Uraemia   D. Toxic goitre
    E. Severe anaemia

Ans.	138. D	139. B	140. D	141. A	142. D	143. D	144. B	145. C	146. C	147. B
	148. D	149. A	150. C	151. A	152. C	153. B	154. A	155. E	156. D	

157. **Which of the following is true regarding handling of gas cylinders:** DNB 1989
A. Don't store in upright position.
B. Don't store in cool place.
C. Don't apply grease to valves repeatedly during storage.
D. Don't close valve when cylinder is empty.

158. **Each gram of haemoglobin can combine with c.c. oxygen :** AIIMS 1985
A. 0.34
B. 1.34
C. 2.34
D. 3.33

159. **Sellick manoeuver :** AIIMS 1987, 97
A. Prevents regurgitation
B. Backward pressure on the cricoid cartilage
C. Backward pressure on hyoid cartilage
D. A and B are correct
E. A and C are correct

160. **The critical temperature of a gas is :** DNB 1989
A. At which it liquifies when pressure is decreased.
B. Above which it will not liquify despite increased pressure.
C. Below which it solidifies.
D. None of the above.

161. **Kussmaul breathing is suggestive of :** Bihar 1989
A. Diabetic alkalosis
B. Renal alkalosis
C. Metabolic alkalosis
D. Respiratory alkalosis

162. **Neurovascular bundle in each intercostal space comprises of :** DNB 1989
A. Posterior Intercostal Vein
B. Posterior Intercostal Artery
C. Intercostal Nerve
D. All of the above
E. None of the above

163. **Tracheal Bifurcation is termed as :** Delhi 1983
A. Angle of Louis
B. Carina
C. Waldeyer's Ring
D. Azygos
E. Vestibular fold

164. **"Tare Weight" term is used in Anaesthetic apparatus for :** AIIMS 1985
A. Gas Cylinders
B. Reservoir Bag
C. Boyle Apparatus as a whole
D. Adapters and connectors

165. **The blood lactate level is elevated in :** AIIMS 1985
A. Severe Metabolic Alkalosis
B. Respiratory Alkalosis
C. Respiratory Acidosis
D. A and B are true
E. B and C are true

166. **The clinical effect of uneven ventilation is :** AIIMS 1985
A. Metabolic alkalosis
B. Respiratory acidosis
C. Hypoxemia
D. CO_2 Retention
E. None of the above

167. **Tracheal tug is associated with :** AIIMS 1986
A. Carbon dioxide narcosis
B. Deep anaesthesia
C. Biphasic block
D. Vasomotor paralysis

168. **Hyperventilation techniques in a anaesthesia result in :** PGI 1987
A. Peripheral vasoconstriction
B. Hypertension
C. Decreases in Lactate/Pyruvate ratio in blood
D. None of the above

169. **Acute tolerance is property of the following drug :** AIIMS 1986
A. Morphine
B. Alcohol
C. Thiopentone
D. Heroin

170. **To prevent static electricity :** AIIMS 1985
A. Use nylon dresses
B. Use cotton dresses
C. Non-conducting floors
D. Rubber matteresses

171. **The Boyle machine is :** AIIMS 1986
A. Continuous flow type
B. Intermittent type
C. Draw over type
D. Temperature compensated type

172. **Arterial hypotension encountered during anaesthesia may be due to which of the following :** AIIMS 1986
A. Vascular absorption of local anaesthetics
B. Surgical manipulation
C. Haemorrhage
D. All of the above

173. **Positive pressure applied to the airway to ventilate the lungs :** PGI 1987
A. Most often causes transient hypertension.
B. Raises cardiac output greatly.
C. Has no effect on blood pressure or circulatory dynamics.
D. May responsible for marked hypotensive.

174. **Platypnea is a feature of :** DNB 1995
A. COPD
B. Bronchial asthma
C. Right to left shunts
D. ASD

Ans.	157. C	158. B	159. D	160. B	161. A	162. D	163. B	164. A	165. D	166. C
	167. B	168. C	169. C	170. B	171. A	172. D	173. A	174. C		

175. Sighing is noted in : **AIIMS 1983**
    A. Light anaesthesia   B. Deep anaesthesia
    C. Both of the above   D. None of the above

176. All of the following differ in males and females except : **Assam 1995**
    A. Tidal volume
    B. Vital capacity
    C. Residual volume
    D. Expiratory reserve volume

177. In Magill's system, air entry is : **AI 1996, 98**
    A. Twice to that of tidal volume
    B. Equal to minute volume
    C. Half of minute volume
    D. One third of tidal volume

178. Spinal cord in neonates terminates at : **Delhi 1985**
    A. D12   B. L2
    C. L3   D. L5

179. Hypotension following spinal anaesthesia requires all the following except : **Bihar 1989**
    A. I/V fluids
    B. Elevation of head end of bed
    C. Vasopressors
    D. O_2 inhalation

180. While giving brachial plexus block, one must do : **AMC 1987**
    A. Turn the head to opposite side.
    B. Depress the ipsilateral shoulder.
    C. Palpate the subclavian artery.
    D. Inject the local anaesthetic 1 cm. above midclavicular point downwards and medially hitting against the Ist rib.
    E. All of the above

181. Which is the narrowest part of laryngeal cavity in adult : **AMC 1989**
    A. Inlet of Larynx   B. Rima Vestibulae
    C. Rima Glottidis   D. Piriform fossa
    E. None of the above

182. All of the following respiratory volumes can be measured by simple spirometre except : **Delhi 1987**
    A. Vital Capacity
    B. Functional Residual Capacity
    C. Tidal Volume
    D. Expiratory Reserve Volume

183. The Surfactant material lining the lung alveoli : **AP 1990**
    A. Is Diapalmitoyl Lecithin.
    B. Type-II cells of Alveolar Epithelium probably give rise to surfactant.
    C. Increases the compliance of lungs.
    D. Decrease the surface tension of alveolar fluid.
    E. All of the above.

184. In chronic Bronchitis and Emphysema all of the following are true except : **DNB 1990**
    A. At rest the rate of O_2 uptake is decreased.
    B. Increased in Residual volume.
    C. VA/Q i.e. ventilation perfusion ratio is a poor indicator of the severity of the disease.
    D. Peak Expiratory flow rate usually reduced.
    E. None of the above.

185. Raised $PaCO_2$ indicates : **DNB 1990**
    A. Alveolar hyperventilation
    B. Bronchial Asthma
    C. Pulmonary fibrosis
    D. Alveolar hypoventilation
    E. Pulmonary arteriovenous fistula

186. Carotid body is not stimulated by : **DNB 1990**
    A. Hypoxic hypoxia   B. Anaemic hypoxia
    C. Stagnant hypoxia   D. Histotoxic hypoxia

187. Cyanosis is absent in : **AIIMS 1987**
    A. Emphysema
    B. Carbon Monoxide poisoning
    C. Polycythaemia
    D. Fallot's tetralogy
    E. Respiratory airways obstruction

188. Which of the following Anaesthetic Apparatus system provides very efficient humidification : **AIIMS 1983**
    A. To and Fro
    B. Non-Rebreathing valve
    C. Ayre T piece
    D. Closed circle absorber

189. All of the following are various methods of humidification of inspired air or gas except : **AIIMS 1985**
    A. Water Bath
    B. Few point hygrometre
    C. Artificial nose with replaceable heat and moisture exchange
    D. Ultrasonic Nebulizer
    E. Mechanical Nebulizer (Bird)

Ans.	175. B	176. D	177. B	178. C	179. B	180. E	181. C	182. B	183. E	184. A
	185. D	186. D	187. B	188. A	189. B					

190. In an unconscious patient, the principle difficulty in maintaining a perfect airways is due to the tendency of :   AIIMS 1984
A. Tongue fall forwards and obstruct the larynx.
B. Tongue fall forward and obstruct the Posterior Nasal opening.
C. Tongue fall backwards and obstruct the posterior nasal opening.
D. Tongue fall forwards and obsfruct the posterior nasal opening.

191. In adults, Anatomically the larynx lies at the level of :   Delhi 1986
A. 2nd to 5th cervical vertebra
B. 3rd to 6th cervical vertebra
C. 4th to 7th cervical vertebra
D. 5th to 8th cervical vertebra
E. None of the above

192. Filum terminale interna which end with the dura and the arachnoid mater at the level of :   UPSC 1986
A. S5 vertebra
B. S2 vertebra
C. S1 vertebra
D. S3 vertebra

193. Number of spinal nerves that emerges from spinal cord in pairs is :   DNB 1989
A. 34
B. 31
C. 57
D. 30

194. Intravertebral foramina number is :   Delhi 1991
A. 59
B. 58
C. 57
D. 60

195. Constituent of "Lytic cocktail" employed to induce hypothermia for vascular or neurosurgery is/are :   Rohtak 1988
A. Promethazine 50 mg
B. Pethidine 100 mg
C. Morphine 30 mg
D. A + B

196. The optimal granule size of soda lime is :   AIIMS 1985
A. 4 to 8 mesh
B. 8 to 10 mesh
C. 10 to 12 mesh
D. 12 to 16 mesh

197. Ether anaesthesia with Schimmelbusch mask is :   TN 1990
A. Open system
B. Semi-open system with non-rebreathing valve
C. Semi-open without valve
D. Close system

198. Magill attachment is a :   Delhi 1985
A. Mapelson A system
B. Mapelson B system
C. Mapelson C system
D. Mapelson D system

199. In intensive care unit, best indicator to measure oxygenation of tissue is :   DNB 1991
A. Capillary PO_2
B. Arterial PO_2
C. Mixed venous oxygen
D. Central venous pressure

200. Pierre Robin syndrome includes :   AIIMS 1986
A. Micrognathia
B. Glossoptosis
C. Cleft palate
D. All of the above

201. Ventilation perfusion ratio is :   DNB 1989
A. 0.5
B. 0.8
C. 1.0
D. 1.2

202. Gastric emptying is increased in :   AIIMS 1986
A. Hypertonic food
B. Hypotonic food
C. Isotonic food
D. None of the above

203. First sign of complication of anaesthesia is :   AI 1990
A. Tachycardia
B. Bradycardia
C. Hypertension
D. Convulsion

204. The critical value of cerebral perfusion pressure is —— mm Hg.   DNB 1993
A. 10-20
B. 30-40
C. 50-60
D. 70-80

205. All of the following are characteristics of pain receptors except that they are not :   DNB 1989
A. Encapsulated receptors
B. Free nerve endings
C. Widespread in arterial walls
D. Widespread in superficial layers of skin

206. Unconscious patients are best nursed in :   Delhi 1983
A. Supine position
B. Lateral position
C. Fowler's position
D. Trendelenburg position

207. Endotracheal intubation is indicated in all except :   AIIMS 1984
A. Short operation with spontaneous breathing.
B. In patients with full stomach.
C. In thoracic and head neck operations.
D. In prone and sitting position.

208. Tracheostomy is indicated in all except :   UPSC 1986
A. Obstruction of air way.
B. Long term artificial ventilation.
C. Unconscious patients in whom pharyngeal reflexes are absent.
D. For aspiration of tracheobronchial tree.

209. Regarding paraldehyde excretion which of the following is true :   AIIMS 1984
A. It is excreted through kidneys
B. It is excreted through sweat glands
C. It is excreted through lungs
D. It is excreted by none of the above means

Ans.	190. C	191. B	192. B	193. B	194. B	195. D	196. A	197. A	198. A	199. B
	200. D	201. B	202. B	203. A	204. B	205. A	206. B	207. A	208. A	209. A

210. Which of the following should not be included in the treatment of hyperkalemia ?   **AP 1989**
  A. Insulin
  B. I/V glucose
  C. Digitalis
  D. I/V calcium

211. O2 consumption in an adult in anaesthetised state is :   **DNB 1990**
  A. 25-50 c.c/square meter/minute
  B. 50-80 c.c/square meter/minute
  C. 80-110 c.c/square meter/minute
  D. 110-130c.c/square meter/minute

212. Which of the following is most effective vasopressor agent ?   **AI 1989**
  A. Adrenaline
  B. Noradrenaline
  C. Angiotensin
  D. Bradykinin
  E. All of the above are equally effective

213. Assessment of patient with cardiac disease includes consideration of the :   **AP 1990**
  A. State of vessel wall
  B. State of myocardium
  C. Condition of the lungs
  D. All of the above

214. Indication of pudendal nerve block may include :   **AMC 1986**
  A. Delayed second stage
  B. Foetal distress
  C. Associated breech delivery
  D. All of the above

215. An increased dose of spinal anaesthesia is indicated in a patient who is :   **DNB 1991**
  A. Obese
  B. Tall
  C. Pregnant
  D. With ascites

216. Following administration of suxamethonium, an increase in serum K+ of ———mmol/L is usually seen: **AIIMS 1985, 89**
  A. 0.1—0.2
  B. 0.2—0.5
  C. 0.5—1.0
  D. 1.5—2.0

217. During phase of inspiration :   **DNB 1989**
  A. Pulse strength increases
  B. Pulse strength decreases
  C. There is no change in pulse strength
  D. All of the above

218. The normal dead space is about :   **AIIMS 1986**
  A. 30% of tidal volume
  B. 40% of tidal volume
  C. 50% of tidal volume
  D. 60% of tidal volume

219. Cyanosis of caused by :   **AIIMS 1986**
  A. Decreased percentage of oxygenated haemoglobin.
  B. Increased percentage of deoxygenated haemoglobin.
  C. Decreased concentration of oxygenated haemoglobin.
  D. Increased concentration of deoxygenated haemoglobin.

220. Which of the following is lighter than air ?   **DNB 1989**
  A. Oxygen
  B. Ethylene
  C. Carbon dioxide
  D. None of the above

221. How much blood is pumped to brain in a normal healthy conscious individual ?   **AIIMS 1984**
  A. Half of total cardiac output
  B. 1/4 th of total cardiac output
  C. 1/6th of total cardiac output
  D. 1/8th of total cardiac output

222. In an adult, normal CSF pressure is :   **UPSC 1984, 86**
  A. 6 mm Hg
  B. 10 mm Hg
  C. 15 mm Hg
  D. 15-20 mm Hg

223. First relay station of pain is :   **Delhi 1984**
  A. Spinal cord
  B. Medulla
  C. Pons
  D. Thalamus

224. First synapse for peripheral sensation is :   **Delhi 1984**
  A. Cerebellum
  B. Anterior horn cells
  C. Posterior horn cells
  D. Mid brain

225. To prevent aspiration of secretions into the trachea, the cuff of the endotracheal tube should be inflated :   **TN 1984**
  A. Above the vocal cord
  B. On the vocal cord
  C. Just below the vocal cord
  D. Inside the bronchus

226. "Sniffing the morning air" position is :   **AIIMS 1985**
  A. Flexion at atlanto-occipital joint and extension of neck.
  B. Flexion of neck with extension of atlanto-occipital joint.
  C. Lateral flexion of neck with flexion of atlanto occipital joint.
  D. Flexion of neck with flexion at atlanto-occipital joint.

227. MAC is :   **DNB 1989**
  A. Maximum air current
  B. Maximum air concentration
  C. Maximum alveolar compression
  D. Minimum alveolar concentration

228. Total body water is :   **AIIMS 1985**
  A. 50% of body weight
  B. 40% of body weight
  C. 60% of body weight
  D. 80% of body weight

Ans.	210. C	211. D	212. C	213. D	214. D	215. B	216. C	217. B	218. A	219. C
	220. B	221. C	222. B	223. A	224. C	225. C	226. B	227. D	228. C	

229. Estimated blood volume for an adult is :
AIIMS 1985
A. 75 ml/kg of body weight
B. 90 ml/kg of body weight
C. 80 ml/kg of body weight
D. 60 ml/kg of body weight

230. Diagnosis of the causes of prolonged Apnoea includes :   AIIMS 1985
A. Electrical stimulation of peripheral nerve
B. PaCO2 and Serum cholinesterase level estimation
C. Edrophonium, to exclude dual block once shallow respiration has commenced
D. Only A and B are true

231. Use of relaxants in Electroconvulsive therapy is termed as :   AIIMS 1984
A. Electric stimulation   B. Electrocution
C. Electropexy   D. Electro motive force
E. Electrolyte imbalance

232. Tissue/Blood solubility coefficient of halothane is greatest in human :   AMU 1988
A. Brain   B. Lung
C. Kidney   D. Fat
E. Muscle

233. Fluotec Vaporizer "Mark III" used for halothane is :   AMU 1986
A. Temperature compensated
B. Flow controlled
C. Pumping effect is eliminated
D. All of the above
E. None of the above

234. Following a single period of tricholorethylene administration , metabolic products are found in the urine from: DNB 1989
A. 2 hour to 24hour   B. 2 days to 4 days
C. 6 days to 12 days   D. 10 days to 18 days
E. 1month to 2 month

235. Blood replacement (Transfusion) is necessary only when the loss is more than: DNB 1989
A. 10% of estimated blood volume
B. 25% of estimated blood volume
C. 15% of estimated blood volume
D. 20% of estimated blood volume

236. 'Supine Hypotensive syndrome' is :   AIIMS 1986
A. Hypotension occurring in supine position
B. Severe hypotension due to prolonged surgery
C. Compression of aorta and vena cava by the gravid uterus when lying supine
D. Hypotensive condition where patient should never be kept in supine position

237. Complication of anaesthesia occurs during :
AIIMS 1986
A. Induction and maintenance
B. Maintenance and recovery
C. Induction and recovery
D. All of the above

238. Mendelson's syndrome is best avoided by :
UPSC 1986
A. Complete starvation of patient
B. Antacid treatment (0.3) Molar sod. citrate) before induction
C. Rapid sequence induction
D. All of the above

239. Incidence of abortion in a pregnant patient due to anaesthesia is high in :   DNB 1989
A. First trimester   B. Second trimester
C. Third trimester   D. All of the above

240. The sciatic nerve in buttock can be located between :   Delhi 1982
A. Ischial tuberosity and lesser trochanter
B. Ischial tuberosity and greater trochanter
C. Ischial tuberosity and iliac crest
D. Ischial tuberosity and coccyx

241. The best way to maintain patent airway in an asphyxiated patient is :   AMC 1983
A. Mouth to mouth breathing
B. Tracheostomy
C. Hyperextension of neck
D. Endotracheal intubation

242. The spinal cord terminates opposite —— vertebra :   TN 1990
A. Lumbar 1st   B. Lumbar 2nd
C. Sacral 1st   D. Sacral 2nd

243. Ventral Rami of which of the following nerves take part in the formation of lumbar plexus ?AIIMS 1988
A. L1 2 3   B. L3 4 5
C. L1 2 3 4   D. L4 5 S1

244. The termination of inner layer of spinal dura is at :   DNB 1989
A. T10   B. T12
C. L2   D. L5
E. S2

245. For immediate post operative airway obstruction, the treatment is :   Delhi 1988
A. Hyper extention of head with elevation of jaw.
B. Tracheostomy.
C. Reintubation.
D. Introduction of oxygen through nose.

Ans.	229. A	230. D	231. C	232. D	233. D	234. D	235. C	236. C	237. C	238. D
	239. A	240. B	241. D	242. A	243. C	244. E	245. A			

246. The following statements are true except :

AP 1989

A. Intrapleural pressure is negative both during expiration and inspiration.
B. I.P.P.V reduces the venous return to heart and cardiac output.
C. I.P.P.V decreases the physiological dead space.
D. Compliance is decreased by I.P.P.V.

247. One of the following is not true :   AP 1989
A. Oxyhaemoglobin curve is S shaped
B. 1.34 ml of oxygen is carried by 1 gm of haemoglobin
C. Shift of the curve is left due to alkalosis and right due to acidosis
D. PO_2 of venous blood is 100 mm of mercury

248. All are true except :   TN 1990
A. 3 to 5% of CO_2 is transported as dissolved CO_2.
B. 13% is carried as carbamino haemoglobin.
C. 82% is carried is bicarbonate.
D. Partial pressure of CO_2 in venous blood is 40 mm of mercury.

249. During deep hypothermia, the brain temperature is measured most accurately in the :   AIIMS 1986
A. Rectum   B. Oesophagus
C. Skin   D. Middle ear

250. Factors which give rise to increased wound bleeding during operation includes all except :   AIIMS 1981
A. Hypercapnia
B. Adequate Analgesia
C. Respiratory obstruction
D. Inhalation anaesthetic agents e.g. Ether and Cyclopropane
E. Improper posture

251. Pre-Capillary vessels in Pulmonary circulations differs from those of systemic circulation is, that in former, they are :   PGI 1987
A. Thick wall   B. Thin wall
C. Easily distensible   D. Both A and C are true
E. Both B and C are true

252. A fall in pulmonary blood volumes occurs in all except :   PGI 1988
A. Left Ventricular failure
B. Valsalva's manoeuvre
C. Assuming upright posture
D. During positive pressure breathing
E. After Haemorrhage

253. Eisenmenger's Complex comprise/s :   DNB 1990
A. Pulmonary Hypertension
B. V.S.D.
C. Right-to-Left Shunt

D. All of the above
E. Only A and B are true

254. Any Vascular connection between the left and right sides of circulations at the atrial, ventricular or aortopulmonary level, causing a right-to-left-shunt is called as :   DNB 1990
A. Fallot's Tetrology
B. Eisenmenger Syndrome
C. Ebstein Anomaly
D. V.S.D. with reversed shunt only
E. None of the above

255. Methods of Measurement of pulmonary blood flow includes all except :   DNB 1990
A. Kety-Schmidt method B. Radio-active Gases
C. Dye-dilution method D. Body plethysmorgraph
E. None of the above

256. Early complications of tracheostomy are :

Bihar 1991

A. Haemorrhage
B. Displacement of tube or obstruction
C. Surgical emphysema
D. Tracheal stenosis

257. Hypoxia causes the following except :   DNB 1991
A. Rise in blood pressure and pulse rate
B. Fall in respiratory rate
C. Restlessness and anxiety
D. Cyanosis

258. Drugs that mimic the responses obtained as a result of stimulation of sympathetic or adrenergic nerves are termed as :   AIIMS 1983
A. Sympathomimetic drugs
B. Sympatholytic drugs
C. Cholinomimetic alkaloids
D. Cholinesterase inhibitors
E. Ganglion stimulating agents

259. Catecholamine content of human adrenal medulla normally is :   AIIMS 1983
A. 50% Adrenaline and 50% of Noradrenaline.
B. 15 % Adrenaline and 85% of Noradrenaline.
C. 85% Adrenaline and 15% of Noradrenaline.
D. 25 % Adrenaline and 75% of Noradrenaline.
E. None of the above.

260. The complication of Hypothermia include/s :

AIIMS 1982

A. Ventricular fibrillation
B. Brain damage
C. Tendency to haemorrhage
D. Frost bite due to local injury
E. All of the above

Ans.	246. C	247. D	248. D	249. D	250. B	251. E	252. A	253. D	254. B	255. A
	256. B	257. B	258. A	259. C	260. E					

261. Uses of Hypothermia in clinical practice are :
AMC 1984
   A. Cardiac Surgery
   B. Neuro Surgery
   C. Operation in great vessels
   D. Treatment of Hyperpyrexia e.g. in thyrotoxic crisis, malignant hyperpyexia etc.
   E. All of the above

262. The major Complications of Extra Corporeal Circulation are : AIIMS 1982
   A. Trauma to formed elements of blood
   B. Air Embolism
   C. Post perfusion lung
   D. All of the above
   E. None of the above

263. The average daily intake of Hydrogen ions, in diet, in the form of sulphur containing amino acids of proteins is : AIIMS 1984
   A. 10-30 mmol/day (mEQ/day)
   B. 30-50 mmol/day (mEQ/day)
   C. 50-80 mmol/day (mEQ/day)
   D. 100-140 mmol/day (mEQ/day)
   E. 500-700 mmol/day (mEQ/day)

264. The sole channel of Hydrogen ion excretion from the body is : DNB 1991
   A. Blood   B. Urine
   C. Sweat   D. Stool
   E. Bile

265. Substances which by their presence in solution increase the amount of acid or alkali which must be added to cuase a unit shift in pH are known as :
AIIMS 1984
   A. Alkalies   B. Buffers
   C. Catalysts   D. All of the above
   E. Only A and C are true

266. ———— pressure refers to the colloid osmotic a solution and is a measure of pressure, usually measure in centimeters of water, generated by plasma proteins of which molecular weight is above 40,000 which do not readily escape through the capillary endothelium:
PGI 1983
   A. Osmotic   B. Oncotic
   C. Hydrostatic   D. Hydraulic
   E. All of the above

267. Anion gap is increased in all of the following conditions except : Delhi 1984, 86
   A. Uraemia   B. Diabetic ketoacidosis
   C. Overhydration   D. Salicylate poisoning
   E. Lactic Acidosis

268. Regarding the fluid and electrolyte into "third space", it : AIIMS 1986
   A. Should be replaced with Ringer lactate solution
   B. Follows extensive soft tissue injuries
   C. Follows perioperative trauma
   D. Follows burns
   E. All of the above

269. All of the following will occur in blood after 7 days of storage except : DNB 1989
   A. Decreased concentration of plasma potassium.
   B. Decreased concentration of platelets.
   C. Decreased concentration of factors, VII, VIII & IX.
   D. Decreased concentration of dextrose and increased concentration of lactic acid.
   E. An increased prothrombin time.

270. One of the pathophysiological effect of IPPV is :
AMU 1990
   A. Decreased cardiac output
   B. Hepatic failure
   C. Poor intestinal function
   D. Pneumothorax

271. Bier's block is : AIIMS 1985
   A. Subaracnoid block
   B. Peripheral nerve block
   C. Infilteration and surface block
   D. Intravenous block

272. For elective cases, the minimum haemoglobin necessary is : AIIMS 1985
   A. 12 gm/dl   B. 10 gm/dl
   C. 9 gm/dl   D. 14 gm/dl

273. To decrease the resistance of airways in children, which of the following is used : AIIMS 1984, 85
   A. Flap valves   B. Inspiratory valves
   C. Expiratory valves D. No valves used

274. In an intensive care unit (ICU), the best indicator to measure oxygenation of tissues is :
AIIMS 1984, 87
   A. Capillary blood   B. Arterial blood
   C. Mixed venous oxygen D. Central venous pressure

275. The fluid of choice in hypovolemic shock is :
AIIMS 1984, 85
   A. Ringer lactate
   B. Low molecular weight dextran
   C. Uncrossed 'O' blood
   D. 5% Dextrose

276. Human body can store oxygen for :
AIIMS 1983, 85
   A. 4—10 minutes   B. 15—20 minutes
   C. 25 minutes   D. 30 minutes

Ans.	261. E	262. D	263. C	264. B	265. B	266. B	267. C	268. E	269. A	270. A
	271. D	272. B	273. D	274. B	275. B	276. A				

277. **Activation of oculo-cardiac reflex frequently occurs during :**   AIIMS 1986, 88
    A. Lid repair
    B. Cataract surgery
    C. Strabismus surgery
    D. Perforating injury of the eye

278. **Beneficial effect of dopamine infusion in management of shock is mainly because it :**   AIIMS 1987, 88
    A. Produces marked increase in total peripheal resistance.
    B. Has strong ionotropic action on heart.
    C. Reduces regional arterial resistance in the kidney.
    D. Has strong chronotropic action on heart.

279. **All show wide Alveolar—Arterial O_2 gradient except :**   AIIMS 1988
    A. Bronchiectasis
    B. ARDS (Acute Respiratory Distress Syndrome)
    C Interstitial fibrosis
    D Central hypoventilation

280. **Acebutolol is contraindicated with all except :**   AIIMS 1985
    A. Morphine
    B. Atropine
    C. Verapamil
    D. Non-deplorazing agents

281. **Acute hypervasulation syndrome causes :**   AIIMS 1988
    A. Decreased $PaCO_2$
    B. Normal PaO_2
    C. Normal or raised HCO_3
    D. Normal or reduced pH

282. **Pyridine-2-Aloxime is drug of choice in :**   AIIMS 1988,89
    A. Organophosphorus poisoning
    B. Endrin poisoning
    C. Barbiturate poisoning
    D. Datura poisoning

283. **True about cardiac temponade except :**   AIIMS 1990
    A. Rapid Y descent   B. Pulsus paradoxus
    C. Kussmaul breathing   D. Electric alternans

284. **DOC in anaphylactic shock due to penicillin is :**   AIIMS 1990
    A. Steroids   B. Adrenaline
    C. Penicillinase   D. Antisera

285. **Neonatal respiratory distress is characterised by :**   AIIMS 1990
    A. Alkalosis (metabolic)   B. Hypercapnia
    C. Hypoglycemia   D. Hypocalcemia

286. **Complication of positive pressure ventillation :**   PGI 1985
    A. Pneumothorax   B. Bradycardia
    C. ↓ ventilation   D. Arrythmias

287. **Central venous pressure (cm of H2O) is :**   PGI 1985
    A. 0-5   B. 5-10
    C. 10-15   D. 15-20

288. **The following are the complications of prolonged endotracheal tube except :**   PGI 1985, 87
    A. Stenosis
    B. Necrosis
    C. Ulceration
    D. Posterior arytenoid paralysis

289. **Hypovolemic shock occurs when intravascular volume is decreased by :**   PGI 1986
    A. 5-10%   B. 15-45%
    C. 45-60%   D. 60-75%

290. **Adrenaline is used in treatment of following except :**   PGI 1984, 87
    A. Shock
    B. Bronchial asthma
    C. Cardiac arrest
    D. Hypersensitivity reaction
    E. Cardiac arrhythmias

291. **All of the following drugs produce hypotension except :**   DNB 1992
    A. Alcuronium   B. Pancuronium
    C. Atracuronium   D. Doxacurium
    E. Mivacurium

292. **Sudden unexpected cardiac arrest occurs in the following except :**   PGI 1987
    A. Ketamine   B. Methohexitone
    C. Lignocaine   D. Cyclopropane
    E. Procaine

293. **In air, the percentage of carbon dioxide is :**   PGI 1988
    A. 4%   B. 0.04%
    C. 0.4%   D. 0.004%

294. **A Patient exposed to chemical industry present with CNS depression, pain chest and excessive lacrimation. probable cause is :**   PGI 1988
    A. Carbon monoxide   B. Methyl isocyanide
    C. Phosgene   D. SO2

295. **if initially succinylcholine produces muscular rigidity, needful is :**   PGI 1989
    A. Increase dose of drug   B. Give pancuronium
    C. Cancel operation   D. Record temperature
    E. Give dentrolene

Ans.	277. D	278. C	279. D	280. B	281. A	282. A	283. A	284. B	285. C	286. A
	287. B	288. D	289. B	290. E	291. B	292. D	293. B	294. B	295. A	

296. Actions of acetylcholine are following except :
    PGI 1989
    A. Dilates pulmonary vasculature
    B. Constricts systemic vsculature
    C. - gastric secretion
    D. Sweating
    E. Diarrhea

297. 100 gm of sodalime absorbs — % of its own weight of CO_2 :
    A. 15   B. 20
    C. 100   D. 150

298. For cyanosis to be manifested, the minimum amount of reduced hemoglobin in blood should be :
    AIIMS 1984
    A. 3 gm%   B. 5 gm%
    C. 8 gm%   D. 10 gm%

299. The decrease in hematocrit is vital if it is :
    AIIMS 1984,85
    A. 40%   B. 25%
    C. 30%   D. 20%

300. In a patient with burns, the best indicator of sufficient perfusion is :   **AIIMS 1984**
    A. Central venous pressure
    B. Hematocrit
    C. Urine output
    D. Hemaglobin concentration

301. Mean pulmonary wedge pressure is :
    AIIMS 1984,85
    A. 5 mm Hg   B. 10 mm Hg
    C 20 mm Hg   C. 25 mm Hg

302. Foetal hemoglobin at birth is what percentage of total hemoglobin :   **AIIMS 1985**
    A. 30%   B. 50%
    C. 70%   D. 90%

303. Cyanosis appears when :
    AIIMS 1985,86; DELHI 1991
    pO2 (mm Hg)   O2 saturation
    A. < 20 mm Hg   < 50%
    B. < 40 mm Hg   < 70%
    C. < 50 mm Hg   < 80%
    D. < 60 mm Hg   < 90%

304. 24 hours excretion of cortisol is approximately :
    AIIMS 1985
    A. 5 mg   B. 10 mg
    C. 20 mg   D. 30 mg

305. Hypothermia is used following except :   **PGI 1998**
    A. Neonatal asphyxia   B. Cardiac surgery
    C. Hyperthermia   D. Arrythmia

306. The site of Ciliary ganglion is :   **PGI 1990**
    A. Optic chiasma .
    B. Apex of orbit lateral to optic nerve.
    C. On lateral rectus.
    D. Lateral orbital wall.
    E. None of the above.

307. High airway resistance in seen in :   **AIIMS 1990**
    A. Respiratory bronchiole
    B. Terminal bronchiole
    C. Intermediate bronchiole
    D. Main bronchus

308. Lumbar puncture is done in the following postion :
    AIIMS 1988
    A. Rt. Lateral
    B. Lt. Lateral
    C. Sitting with head below flexed knees
    D. All of the above

309. Modified Glasgow coma scale defines neurolgoic impairment by the following yardsticks :
    AIIMS 1986
    A. Sensory, motor function and speech
    B. Cardiovascular status, motor function and speech
    C. Pupillary size, motor function and level of consciousness
    D. Eye opening, motor functions and best verbal response

310. Which of the following should not be used in cholinergic crisis: **PGI 1984**
    A. Atropine   B. Ephedrine
    C. Pralidoxime   D. IV Tensilon

311. Pralidoxime acts in organosphorus poisoning by :   **PGI 1986**
    A. Regenerating cholinesterase
    B. Inhibiting cholinesterase
    C. Cholinergic action
    D. All of the above

312. Breur Lockard reflex is :   **PGI 1982**
    A. Reflex hypotension due to pooling in spinal anaesthesia.
    B. Penile engorgement due to spinal anaesthesia.
    C. Reflex bronchospasm due to parasympathetic stress at a different site.
    D. Tracheal tug.

313. High positive pressure respiration causes all except :   **Delhi 1988**
    A. Tracheomalacia   B. Fluid retention
    C. Cerebral oedema   D. O_2 intoxication

Ans.	296. B	297. B	298. B	299. D	300. C	301. B	302. C	303. B	304. C	305. D
	306. B	307. D	308. D	309. D	310. D	311. A	312. C	313. D		

314. Causes of hypercapnia in anaesthetic practice may include :   AIIMS 1982
A. Defective soda lime in faulty circuit
B. Apnoeic insufflation of oxygenation
C. Profound narcosis
D. Muscle relaxants
E. All of the above

315. Minimum rebreathing occus with :   Delhi 1988
A. Rubin valve   B. Leigh valve
C. Open drop method   D. Ayre's technique
E. High flow insufflation

316. All of the following are usually associated with rewarming shock, except :   AIIMS 1984
A. Respiratory acidosis B. Shivering
C. Vasoconstriction   D. Low pH
E. Rapid rewarming

317. Elective surgery in a patient who had a myocardial infarction is best done after :   AIIMS 1983
A. 2 months   B. 3 months
C. 5 months   D. 6 months

318. Endotracheal tubes are sterilised by :   AIIMS 1982
A. Gamma rays   B. Boiling
C. Autoclaving   D. ETO gas

319. The pressure required to inflate the cuff on an endotracheal tube is :   AIIMS 1983
A. 5-10 mm Hg   B. 15-25 mm Hg
C. 30-45 mm Hg   D. 50-60 mm Hg

320. The receptors of pain are :   PGI 1983,85
A. Ruffini organs   B. Merkel's bodies
C. Golgi bodies   D. Free nerve endings

321. On Glasgow coma scale, maximum rating is given to :   DNB 1991
A. Spontaenously opening of eyes
B. Obeying motor command
C. Oriented and converses
D. Opening of eyes to verbal command

322. Bretylium interfers with the release of :
                                        PGI 1982, 84
A. Adrenaline   B. Nor adrenaline
C. DOPA   D. Dopamine

323. The appropriate gauge of endotracheal tube for a 5-6 lb infant is :   AMC 1985
A. 10-12   B. 13-14
C. 17-18   D. 22-23

324. The average distance from the central incisors to the glottis in an adult is about :   Delhi 1987
A. 4-6 cm   B. 8-10 cm
C. 12-14 cm   D. 18-20 cm

325. A vasoconstrictor should not be used for nerve block of :   AIIMS 1982
A. Toe   B. Nose
C. Penis   D. Finger
E. All of the above

326. Van tint's technique is used for blocking : Delhi 1882
A. Fifth cranial nerve   B. Facial nerve
C. Third cranial nerve   D. Fourth cranial nerve
E. None of the above

327. Average intravenous dose of digoxin for emergency digitalization is :   UPSC 1988
A. 0.2 mg   B. 0.4 mg
C. 0.8 mg   D. 1.0 mg
E. 2.0 mg

328. An anaesthesist is worried about: Delhi 1986
A. Bradycardia   B. Hypotension
C. Repeated ectopics D. Tachycardia

329. Nicotinic effects of acetylcholine are blocked by:
                                            Delhi 1986
A. Atropine   B. d-tubocurare
C. Suxamethonium.   D. Magnesium chloride

330. Most common post operative complication is :
                                UPSC 1985; DELHI 1986
A. Aspiration pneumonia B. Lobar pneumonia
C. Seizures   D. Atelectasis

331. While doing a phrenic nerve block, it is the best to infiltrate: PGI 1981
A. Scalenus anticus
B. Scalenus posterior
C. 8th cervical transverse process
D. Anterior border of sternomastoid
E. Posterior border of sternomastoid

332. In a maxillary block, the petrygoid procss of the sphenoid should be reached at :   AIIMS 1980
A. 0.5 cm   B. 6 cm
C. 21 cm   D. 1 cm
E. None of the above

333. Pulmonary function differing in infant compared with adult :   AIIMS 1981
A. Tidal volume F.R.C
B. O2 uptake/minute/kg
C. Respiratory quotient
D. Ventilation/ml O2 uptake
E. Functional residual capacity/kg

334. Most sensitive to specific relaxant drug action :
                                            PGI 1981
A. Diaphragm   B. Arm muscles
C. Neck muscles   D. Abdominal muscles
E. Intercostals

Ans.	314. E	315. E	316. A	317. D	318. B	319. B	320. D	321. B	322. B	323. B
	324. C	325. E	326. B	327. D	328. C	329. B	330. A	331. A	332. B	333. B
	334. C									

335. Breath sound audible for more than——seconds on auscultation over the trachea during forced expiration denotes airways obstruction :

AIIMS 1981

A. 2
B. 4
C. 6
D. 8

336. In the match test, the distance between the lighted paper match and the mouth should be ———cm :

PGI 1981

A. 10
B. 15
C. 20
D. 25

337. The holding below ——indicates lack of cardio-respiratory reserve :

AIIMS 1982

A. 8 seconds
B. 10 seconds
C. 15 seconds
D. 18 seconds
E. 20 seconds

338. Drug which is contraindicated in head injury:

AIIMS 1987

A. Oxygen
B. IV Fluids
C. Morphine
D. Antibiotics

339. In incubator, heat is delivered by following except :

PGI 1998

A. Conduction
B. Convection
C. Radiation
D. Evaporation

340. The placenta is readily permeable to :

AIIMS 1982; DNB 1988

A. C_3H_6
B. Mepindine
C. Ether
D. Barbiturates
E. All of the above

341. In case of CPR, following is true :   AIIMS 1998

A. I/V adrenatine should be given if fibrillator fails
B. Asystole characteristic finding in ECG
C. In 2 persons, CPR ratio is 5 : 1
D. I/V calcium, gluconate is given immediately

342. Dead space is decreased by all except :   DNB 1988

A. Tracheostomy
B. Lifting jaw forward
C. Supine position
D. Intubation
E. All of the above

343. Blood pressure during anaesthesia is monitored by:

Delhi 1998

A. Femoral artery
B. Temporal artery
C. Radial artery
D. Ulnar artery
E. All of the above are true

344. Contraindications to induced hypotension :

PGI 1981

A. Pulmonary oedema
B. Low blood pressure
C. History of myocardial infarct
D. History of cerebral thrombosis
E. None of the above

345. Capnography is :   Delhi 1998

A. Monitoring of concentration of exhaled CO_2
B. Monitoring of concentration of inhaled O_2
C. Monitoring of blood pressure during anaesthesia .
D. Monitoring of central venous pressure

346. Anatomical dead space is increased by following except :   AI 1999

A. Massive pleural effusion
B. Inspiration
C. Atropine
D. Halothane

347. Compliance of lungs and thorax is reduced in :

UPSC 1982

A. General anaesthesia
B. Kyphoscoliosis
C. Poliomyelitis
D. Congestive cardiac failure
E. All of the above

348. Tachycardia should be avoided in all of the following except :   AIIMS 1986

A. Aortic stenosis
B. Mitral stenosis
C. Coronary artery disease
D. Mitral regurgitation

349. One of the following is contraindicated in pulmonary oedema :   AIIMS 1986

A. Morphine
B. Trendelenburg position
C. IPPV
D. Antitrendelenburg position

350. A lower heart rate is beneficial in :   DNB 1990

A. Constrictive pericarditis
B. Cardiac tamponade
C. Mitral stenosis
D. Aortic regurgitation

351. Heart block can result because of surgery in patients with :   DNB 1991

A. ASD
B. PDA
C. Coarctation
D. VSD

352. Following are semiopen circuits except :

AIIMS 1985

A. Magill's
B. Mapelson E
C. Magill with non rebreathing value
D. Ayre's T piece

Ans.	335. C	336. B	337. C	338. C	339. D	340. E	341. C	342. B	343. C	344. E
	345. A	346. A	347. E	348. D	349. B	350. C	351. D	352. D		

353. Early sign of respiratory obustruction is :

Karnataka 1987

A. Cyanosis
B. Retraction of chest wall
C. Noisy breathing
D. Excessive abdominal movement

354. Anaesthetic induction in children is by : AIIMS 1993

A. Inhalation
B. IV
C. IM
D. Perrectal

355. Oxygen delivery is regulated by all except :

AIIMS 1993

A. Noval catheter
B. Venti mask
C. Poly mask
D. Oxygen tent

356. The purpose of cuff of endotracheal tube in anaesthesia is:

Delhi 1994

A. Provide airtight seal in trachea
B. Prevents dislocation
C. Avoiding damage to trachea
D. All of the above

357. In a patient starts getting convlsions following the use of lignocaine as local anaesthetic the drug of choice for the control of convulsions would be :

UPSC 1994

A. Diazepam
B. Scoline
C. Chlorpromazine
D. Any of the above

358. Hyperbaric local anaesthesia used for spinal anaesthesia is :

AI 1994

A. 5% xylocaine
B. 2% xylocaine with dextrose
C. 5% xylocaine with dextrose
D. 2% Bupivacanine

359. Subarachnoid space ends at :

AI 1994

A. L1
B. L2
C. L5
D. S2

360. In mouth to mouth respiration, oxygen supply is :

AI 1994, 96

A. 16%
B. 30%
C. 42%
D. 48%

361. The number of Endotracheal tube respresents :

PGI 1993

A. Internal diameter of the tube in mm
B. External diameter of the tube in mm
C. Internal and external diameter tube in mm
D. Inner diameter of tube in mm

362. Myocardial oxygen demand is maximally increased by :

PGI 1993, 94

A. Halothane
B. Ether
C. TCE
D. N2O

363. In-Ayer's T-tube, ventilation is done at— ml/min/Kg :

PGI 1993,94

A. 60
B. 100
C. 500
D. 1000

364. In external cardiac massage, the sternum must be depressed by :

PGI 1994

A. 1-1.5 inches
B. 1.5-2 inches
C. 2-2.5 inches
D. 4-5 inches

365. Rapid adaptation occurs in the following sensation :

A. Touch
B. Pain
C. Temperature
D. Taste

366. For epidural anaesthesia in a pregnant woman, xylocaine required in comparison to normal is :

PGI 1994

A. 35% more than normal
B. 25% more than normal
C. 15% more than normal
D. 35% more than normal

367. What percentage of trichloroethylene is required for analgesia purpose in labour :

PGI 1994

A. 1.5%
B. 2.5%
C. 3.5%
D. 5%

368. Anuria is called when the urine output is less than—in 24 hours :

PGI 1994

A. 100 ml
B. 200 ml
C. 300 ml
D. 500 ml

369. Specific therapy in treatement of poisoning with anti-CHE include :

PGI 1994

A. Atropine
B. Physostigmine
C. Pralidoxine
D. Adrenaline

370. Regarding rebreathing prevention valves, which is incorrect :

AIIMS 1994

A. Installed at the expiratory end of tube.
B. Should be as far as possible from the patients.
C. Should be light.
D. Suitably designed.

371. All included in clearing airway except :

AIIMS 1995

A. Head lift
B. Chin lift
C. Mouth lift
D. Neck lift

372. Dose of epinephrine required for resuscitation through endotracheal tube is :

Delhi 1995

A. Same as S/C
B. 1.5 times
C. 2.5 times
C. 3.5 times

373. Dose of propofol for induction per Kg is——mg :

Delhi 1995

A. 1
B. 2
C. 4
D. 9

Ans.	353. C	354. A	355. B	356. A	357. A	358. C	359. D	360. A	361. A	362. A
	363. B	364. B	365. A	366. D	367. C	368. A	369. C	370. B	371. D	372. B
	373. B									

374. Gas which contribute to Greenhouse effect is :

Delhi 1995

A. N_2O
B. CO and N_2O
C. CO_2 and N_2O
D. CO_2 and N_2
E. Ozone and CO

375. Spontaneous release of ACh at NM produces :

AI 1995

A. Miniature end plate potentials
B. Action potential
C. Resting membrance potential
D. Post tetanic potentiation

376. Which one of the following interspinous spaces is not considered safe for lumbar puncture ?   UPSC 1995

A. Between first and second lumbar spines
B. Between second and third lumbar spines
C. Between third and fourth lumbar spines
D. Between fourth and fifth lumbar spines

377. A complication of extrathecal morphine is :

PGI 1994, 95

A. Itching
B. hypotension
C. Vomiting
D. Delayed resp. depression

378. The physical law governing cooling at the tip of the cryoprobe goes by the name of: AP 1990

A. Bernoulli
B. Joules-Thompson
C. Venturi
D. Pascal

379. The following drug is used in hypotensive anaesthesia: AP 1991,95

A. Propranolol
B. Sodium nitroprusside
C. Furesemide
D. All of the above

380. Ventilatory support is indicated in all except: AP 1991

A. 40-60 ml/Kg body wt. of vital capacity
B. Respiratory rate 33/min
C. PaO2 is less than 60 mm Hg & PaCo2 60 mm Hg
D. ARDS

381. Swan-Ganz catheter is placed in pulmonary artery can be used for direct measurement of all the following except :   AP 1991

A. CVP
B. Right venticular pressure
C. Left ventricular end diastolic pressure
D. Mixed venous blood gas analysis

382. Improvement of tissue oxygenation in traumatized patients is best attained by the infssion of : AP 1992

A. Bicarbonate
B. Frozen erythrocytes
C. Free haemoglobin
D. Free myoglobin

383. Regarding 'shock lung' all are true except :

AP 1993

A. Decreased lung compliance.
B. Very common major trauma.
C. Microthrombus in pulmonary vessels.
D. Decreased difusion capacity.

384. All of the following are major events in basic life support except :   AP 1995

A. Maintenance of airway
B. External cardiac message
C. Adrenaline
D. Administration of I.V fluids

385. The only tissue where NAD and NADP are equally disturbed :   DELHI 1993,94

A. Bone marrow
B. Liver
C. Kidney
D. Heart

386. In acute blood loss, blood volume is monitored by :

AI 1996

A. CVP
B. Urine output
C. Pulse rate
D. BP

387. Oxygen concentration in anaesthesia is :

Delhi 1996

A. 16%
B. 33%
C. 45%
D. 67%

388. In Magill's system, air entry is :   AI 1996, 98

A. Twice to that of tidal volume
B. Equal to minute volume
C. Half of minute volume
D. One third of tidal volume

389. Following are examples of autocoid antagonists except :   Rajasthan 1994

A. Captopril— peptide dipeptidase
B. Ibuprofen—cyclo oxygenase
C. Prednisolone-phospholipase
D. Hydraallazine cystathione synthetase

390. All are true about PEEP except :   PGI 1999

A. Useful in situations where PO2 is low
B. ↓ CO
C. Impaired renal function
D. ↓ ICT

391. Mismatched blood tranfusion during surgery is manifested as :   PGI 1999

A. ↑ Bleeding
B. Tachycardia
C. Dyspnoea
D. - BP

392. First step to be taken in a case of multiple injuries :

PGI 1999

A. Whole body CT
B. Maintain airway
C. X-ray skull
D. Urgent USG

Ans.	374. C	375. A	376. A	377. B	378. B	379. B	380. B	381. B	382. B	383. C
	384. D	385. B	386. A	387. B	388. B	389. D	390. D	391. A	392. B	

393. A 2 year old child with intercostal retraction and increasing cyanosis was brought with a history of foreign-body aspiration. Which might be lifesaving in this situation :   AIIMS 1999
   A. Oxygen through face mask
   B. Heimlich's manoeuvre
   C. Extra-cardiac massage
   D. Intracardia adrenaline

394. Bag and mask ventilation is absolutely contraindicated in all except :   AIIMS 1999
   A. Tracheo-esophageal fistula with esophageal stresia and esophagus connected to trachea
   B. Diaphragmatic hernia
   C. Meconium aspiration
   D. Multicentric bronchogenic cyst

395. Epinephrine in CPR acts by :   AIIMS 1999
   A. Increased myocardial O2
   B. Increased SA node activity
   C. Peripheral vasoconstriction directing flow to heart
   D. Ratio of epi. cardium blood flow to that of endocardium decreased

396. Expert manoever in CPR, to maintain Airway in well equipped centre :   AIIMS 1999
   A. Endotracheal intubation
   B. Nasopharyngeal Airway
   C. Tracheostomy
   D. Ambu's bag

397. True about post spinal hypotention is all except :   MAHE 1999
   A. Paralysis of nerve supply from
   B. Leakage of CSF through puncture site
   C. Trendelenberg position is good
   D. Elevation of lower limbs without head low position is useful

398. Posttussive suction is characteristic of :   MAHE 1999
   A. Bronchiectasis   B. Pleural effusion
   C. Tubercular cavity   D. Interstitial lung disease

399. Doxapram is a ——— drug :   TN 1999
   A. Respiratory stimulant   B. Antiepileptic
   C. Sedative   D. Anti diabetic

400. Best indicator of CPR is :   AP 1999
   A. Reacting pupil   B. ↑HR
   C. - Carotid pulses   D. ↑ Skin colour

401. Anaesthetic gases are stable in cylinders made of :   AI-2000
   A. Molybdenum steel
   B. Copper iron alloy
   C. Iron
   D. Copper aluminium alloy

402. Size of vapours (aerolised) in humidification is :   AI 2000
   A. 5 microns   B. 10 microns
   C. 100 microns   D. 200 microns

403. Fresh gas flow in a Magill circuit is how many times minute ventilation :   AI 2000
   A. Equal   B. Half
   C. Thrice   D. Four times

404. True about Newtonian fluid is :   AI-2000
   A. Viscosity is proportional to shear stress.
   B. Viscosity is inversally proportional to shear stress.
   C. Viscosity is square of sphear stress.
   D. There is no relationship.

405. Mallampatti test is :   AI 2000
   A. To assess airway patency
   B. To test movements of atlanto occipital joint
   C. To test movements at cervical vertebrae
   D. To test for ventilatory sufficiency in thoracic injury

406. Consider the following statements :
   In the case of cardiopulmonary arrest, the difference in resuscitative measures between an infant and an adult lies in the :   UPSC 2000
   1. Site of sternal compressions.
   2. Depth of sternal compressions
   3. Number of breaths per minute
   4. DC counter shock.
   Which of the above statements are correct ?
   A. 1 and 2   B. 2, 3 and 4
   C. 1, 2, 3 and 4   D. 1, 3 and 4

407. A patient has "street fit" after general anaesthena on OPD basis.The anaesthetie is: JIPMER 2000
   A. Propofol   B. Midazolam
   C. Alfentanyl   D. Thiopentone

408. Isobaric oxygen is used in :   IAM-2000
   A. Respiratory muscle paralysis
   B. Diver's bends
   C. CCF
   D. Gas gangrene

409. In emergency caesarean section, sequence induction is done :   JIPMER 2000
   A. To prevent aspiration
   B. To prevent fetal distress
   C. For easy intubation
   D. To prevent caval compression

Ans.	393. B	394. D	395. B	396. A	397. A	398. C	399. A	400. D	401. A	402. A
	403. A	404. A	405. A	406. C	407. A	408. C	409. C			

410. Sphenoid wing dysplasia is associated with :
    JIPMER 2000
    A. Sturge Weber syndrome
    B. Von Hipple Lindau disease
    C. Tuberous sclerosis
    D. Treacher Collins syndrome

411. In myaesthenia gravis, which is not effective :Delhi 2000
    A. Succinylcholine   B. Neostigmine
    C. Steroids   D. Cyclosporine

412. End-tidal Co2 volume is increased to maximum level in :   **PGI 2000**
    A. Pul. embolism
    B. Malignant hyperthermia
    C. Extubation
    D. Blockage of secretion

413. Hypothermia is used in which surgery :   **PGI 2000**
    A. Fever
    B. Prolonged surgeries
    C. Massive blood transfusion
    D. Hypertension

414. Ca2+ channel blockers in anesthesia. True is :
    PGI 2000
    A. Needs to be decreased as they augment hypotension & muscle relaxation
    B. Withheld because they lower LES pressure
    C. Should be given in normal dose as they prevent MI & angina
    D. All of the above

415. The ideal route of administration of adrenaline in Cardiopulmonary resuscitation is :   **TNPSC 1995**
    A. Intracardiac   B. Intravenous
    C. Intramuscular   D. Intraperitoneal

416. Oxygen inspiration is maximum in :   **UP 1999**
    A. Light face mask   B. Endotracheal tube
    C. Nasal mask   D. Nasal canula

417. Oxyten therapy in "fixed performens" is given with :
    UP 2000
    A. Polymask   B. Ventimask
    C. MC-mask   D. Nasal catheter

418. Serum cortisol level is decreased with :   **UP 2000**
    A. Thiopentone   B. Propofol
    C. Etomidate   D. Methahexitone

419. 5 years old child going for sitting craniotomy, while positioning in O.T. developed end tidal CO2 —zero mm Hg, PO2—80 mm Hg implies :   **AIIMS 2000**
    A. Endotracheal tube in oesophagus
    B. Endotracheal tube blocked with secretions
    C. Venous air embolism
    D. Left lung collapse

420. After hyperventilating for some time, holding the breath is dangerous since :   **AIIMS 2000**
    A. It can lead on to CO_2 narcosis.
    B. Due to the lack of sitmulation by CO_2 anoxia can go into dangerous levels.
    C. Decreased CO_2 shift the oxygen dissociation curve to the left.
    D. Alkalosis can lead on to tetany.

421. All of the following anaesthetic agents can be given in children except :   **AI 2001**
    A. Halothene   B. Ether
    C. Morphine   D. Clonazepam

422. In ARSD, PEEP in ventilators is useful in following except :   **AI 2001**
    A. Increased resorption of fluid
    B. Decreased alveolar collapse
    C. Decreased alveolar fluid accumulation
    D. Prevents barotrauma

423. A.S.A. (American Society of Anaesthesiaologists) classifies patients according to :   **Rajasthan 2001**
    A. Their general condition
    B. Mortility
    C. Morbidity
    D. None

424. Normal value of PaO2 (torr) in preterm infants is :
    Delhi 2001
    A. 70 ± 11   B. 95 ± 8
    C. 93 ±10   D. 60 ± 8

425. Contraindication to laryngeal mask airway is :
    Delhi 2001
    A. Difficult airway
    B. Large tongue
    C. Increased risk of gastric regurgitation
    D. Low air way resistance

426. Route of administration for patient controlled analgesia is :   **Delhi 2001**
    A. Oral   B. Epidural
    C. Intravenous   D. Intramuscular

427. Post spinal hypotension in obstetrics patients is treated by :   **Delhi 2001**
    A. Dopamine infusion
    B. Adrenaline subcutaneously
    C. Crystalloid infusion
    D. Dobutamine infusion

Ans.	410. D	411. A	412. A	413. B	414. A	415. A	416. B	417. D	418. C	419. C
	420. B	421. C	422. D	423. A	424. C	425. C	426. D	427. C		

428. Most common cause of hypoxemia in immediate post operative period is : **Delhi 2001**
A. Low FiO_2
B. Hyperventilation
C. Decreased metabolism
D. Hypoventilation

429. Anatomical dead space is : **Delhi 2001**
A. 50 ml
B. 150 ml
C. 250 ml
D. 350 ml

430. Most fatal complication in anesthesia is : **MAHE 2001**
A. Hypothermia
B. Porphyria
C. Both
D. None

431. Best method to measure the position of endotracheal tube in trachea : **JIPMER 2002**
A. Auscultahon of chest
B. Absence of gurgling sound in epigastrium
C. End tidal CO_2
D. Pulse oximetry

432. Delivery of hypoxic mixtures can be prevented by all except : **JIPMER 2002**
A. Pin index
B. Pressure gauge
C. Low O2 alarm
D. Proportional delivery system

433. In a patient with fixed respiratory obstruction Helium is used along with Oxygen instead of plain oxygen because : **AI 2002**
A. It increases the absorption of oxygen
B. It decreases turbulance
C. It decreases the dead space
D. For analgesia

434. The gas which produces systemic toxicity without causing local irritation is : **AI 2002**
A. Ammonium
B. Carbon monoxide
C. Hydrocyanic acid
D. Sulfur dioxide

435. In cardio-pulmonary resuscitation, when a single person is doing both, ventilation & chest compression, then the ratio of chest compression to ventilation should be : **A.P. 2002**
A. 8 : 2
B. 10 : 2
C. 12 : 2
D. 15 : 2

436. Which of the following is device used for oxygen therapy? **Maharashtra -2002**
A. Pulse oximeter
B. Nickname's catheter
C. Hudson's mask
D. Guedel's airway

437. A 5-year old child is scheduled for strabismus (squint) correction. Induction of anaesthesia is uneventful. After conjunctival incision as the surgeon grasps the medial rectus, the anaesthesiologist looks at the cardiac monitor. Why do you think he did that : **AIIMS 2002**
A. He wanted to check the depth of anaesthesia.
B. He wanted to be sure that the blood pressure did not fall.
C. He wanted to see if there was an oculocardiac reflex.
D. He wanted to make sure there were no ventricular dysthythmias which normally accompany incision.

438. In volume-cycled ventilation, the inspiratory flow rate is set at : **AIIMS 2002**
A. 140-160 L/min.
B. 110-130 L/min.
C. 60-100 L/min.
D. 30-50 L/min.

439. An anaesthetist orders a new attendant to bring the oxygen cylinder. He will ask the attendant to identify the correct cylinder by following color code : **AI 2003**
A. Black cylinder with white shoulders
B. Black cylinder with grey shoulders
C. White cylinder with black shoulders
D. Grey cylinder with white shoulders

440. A 5 yr old boy suffering from Duchenne muscular dystrophy has to undergo tendon lengthening procedure. The most appropriate anaesthetic would be : **AI 2003**
A. Induction with intravenous thiopentone and N_2O, and halothane for maintenance.
B. Induction with intravenous propofol and N_2O and oxygen for maintenance.
C. Induction with intravenous suxamethonium and N_2O; halothane for maintenance.
D. Inhalation inductin with inhalation halothane and N_2O; oxygen for maintenance.

441. A 25 yrs old male is undergoing incision and drainage of abscess under general anaestesia with spontaneous respiration. The most efficient anaesthetic circuit is : **AI 2003**
A. Maplesen A
B. Maplesen B
C. Maplesen E
D. Maplesen D

442. A 64 yr old hypertensive obese female was undergoing surgery for fracture femur under general anaesthesia. Intraoperatively her end tidal carbondioxide decreased to 20 from 40 mm Hg, followed by hypotension and oxygen saturation of 85 %. What could be the most probable cause : **AI 2003**
A. Fat embolism
B. Hypovolemia
C. Bronchospasm
D. Myocardial infarction

Ans.	428. D	429. B	430. A	431. C	432. A	433. B	434. B	435. D	436. C	437. C
	438. D	439. A	440. B	441. A	442. A					

443. A 25 year old male with roadside accident underwent debridement and reduction of fractured both bones right forearm under axillary block. On the second post-operative day the patient complained of persistent numbness and paraesthesia in the right forearm and the hand. The commonest cause of this neurological dysfunction could be all of the following except?
             AI 2004
A. Crush injury to the hand and lacerated nerves.
B. A tight cast or dressing.
C. Systemic toxicity of local anaesthetics.
D. Tourniquet pressure.

444. A lower Segment Caesarean Section (LSCS) canbe carried out under all the following techniques of anaesthesia except :   **AI 2005**
A. General anaesthesia
B. Spinal anaesthesia
C. Caudal anaesthesia
D. Combiend Spinal Epidural anaesthesia

445. Which one of the following anaesthetic agents causes a rise in the Intracranial pressure :   **AI 2005**
A. Sevoflurane   B. Thiopentone sodium
C. Lignocaine   D. Propofol

446. The most appropriate circuit for ventilating a spontaneonsly breathing infant during anaesthesia is :   **AI 2005**
A. Jackson Rees' modificatin of Ayres' T Piece.
B. Mapleson A or Magill's circuit.
C. Mapelson C or Water to and fro canister.
D. Bains circuit.

447. The following modes of ventilation may be used for weaning off patints from mechanical ventilation except :   **AI 2005**
A. Controled Mechanical ventilation (CMV).
B. Synchronized intermittent mandatory ventilation (SIMV).
C. Pressure support ventilation (PSV).
D. Assist - control ventilation (ACV).

448. The laryngeal mask airway used for securing the airway of a patient in all of the following conditions except :   **AI 2005**
A. In a difficult intubation.
B. In cardiopulmonary resuscitation.
C. In a child undergoing an elective/routine eye surgery.
D. In a patient with a large tumor in the oral cavity.

449. Mapleson's classification of anaesthetic breathing systems :   **Karnataka 2005**
A. Describes four systems : A,B,C,D
B. Classifies the Bain system as maples on D.
C. Describes the T-piece as mapleson D.
D. Describes the T-piece system as requiring a fresh gas flow rate of 1.5-2 times

450. Depression of level of consciousness in hyperthermia starts when the core body temperature is below :   **COMEDK-2005**
A. 36 degrees C   B. 34 degrees C
C. 33 degrees C   D. 32 degrees C

Ans.	443. C	444. C	445. A	446. A	447. D	448. D	449. B	450. C

EXPLANATIONS OF MISCELLANEOUS

1. Ans. — D. Frontal headache
2. Ans. — A. LTB$_4$
3. Ans. — C. Guanethidine
4. Ans. — A. The intratracheal administration of mucolytic agents.
5. Ans. — A. Ketamine
6. Ans. — A. Propanidid
    It is a barbiturate metabolized in liver.
7. Ans. — D. Mapelson D system
8. Ans. — C. Venturi mask
9. Ans. — D. Acupunture
10. Ans. — D. 2
11. Ans. — E. Only B and C are true
12. Ans. — C. Heat causes cerebral vasoconstriction while cold has the reverse effect.
13. Ans. — D. Standing
14. Ans. — C. Sitting
15. Ans. — C. Foetal asphyxia
16. Ans. — B. Age
17. Ans. — C. Brown Fat
18. Ans. — B. Cleft Palate
19. Ans. — A. 240 ml
20. Ans. — D. All of the above
21. Ans. — A. 0.5 ATA
22. Ans. — D. Propranolol
23. Ans. — A. Lowest of the three cervical ganglion with the first thoracic ganglion.
24. Ans. — B. Sixth cervical vertebra
25. Ans. — A. Vasoconstrictor
    Felypressin or Octopressin is a synthetic derivative of vasopressin. It causes contraction of all smooth muscles including coronaries but has little oxytoxic or ADH effect. On injection causes local vasoconstriction without secondary vasodilatation as adrenaline does. Available in combination with prilocaine to prolong the effects and increase the efficiency of dental analgesia.

26. Ans. — D. Hypothermia
27. Ans. — A. 4% 95% 1%
28. Ans. — D. Sweating
29. Ans. — B. Unrecognised chest injury
30. Ans. — A. Thiopentone
    Thiopentone reaches maximum concentration in fetal blood very soon after injection into the mother. T-half of distribution phase is 3 min.
31. Ans. — C. Yokes
32. Ans. — A. Wastage of expensive agent and atmospheric pollution
33. Ans. — C. 5
34. Ans. — B. It accomplishes gas exchange without bulk air exchange.
35. Ans. — E. None of the above
36. Ans. — E. Precordial Doppler monitoring
    Air embolism was first reported in 1821 by Magendie and by Barlow in 1830. The factors of importance are volume of air speed of injection, pressure in veins, posture and general condition of patient.
37. Ans. — C. Properly timed atrial contractions
38. Ans. — D. The avoidance or immediate treatment of tachycardia.
39. Ans. — B. Salt-poor albumin
40. Ans. — C. Both of the above
41. Ans. — A. Sitting
42. Ans. — E. All of the above
43. Ans. — C. Neuro Surgical Anaesthesia
44. Ans. — E. All of the above
45. Ans. — B. Rising end expiratory CO$_2$
    Endtidal CO$_2$ fall rapidly if blood does not reach the lungs.
46. Ans. — D. The presence of post-tetanic facilitation
47. Ans. — D. Atropine
48. Ans. — C. Because of its rate of impulse formation
49. Ans. — B. A decrease in the rate of discharge of the AV node.

50. Ans. — B. Between 40% and 45%
51. Ans. — D. The large veins
52. Ans. — C. The capillaries
53. Ans. — E. Monitor ascending spinal tracts during scoliosis surgery.
54. Ans. — C. Pre-capillary resistance
55. Ans. — D. 2.5
56. Ans. — A. High Renin Hypertension

    Propranolol decrease the renin levels.
57. Ans. — B. Sinus Tachycardia
58. Ans. — D. All of the obove
59. Ans. — E. All of the obove
60. Ans. — E. Thoracic aorta surgery
61. Ans. — B. 10° to 15°
62. Ans. — D. Middle ear (tympanic membrane)
63. Ans. — D. Belladonna alkaloids

    It is also common with barbiturates.
64. Ans. — B. Spinal anaesthesia
65. Ans. — B. Primarily a beta agonist
66. Ans. — B. 4.5 mm
67. Ans. — D. Alveolar hypoventilation
68. Ans. — B. 30 mm Hg
69. Ans. — B. There are varying degrees of acute and chronic respiratory insufficiencies.
70. Ans. — E. 6.0 mL
71. Ans. — D. Elevate the head of the bed by 30°.
72. Ans. — D. 7.36
73. Ans. — A. 40 mm Hg
74. Ans. — A. pCO_2 rises, Plasma bicarbonate rises, pH falls.
75. Ans. — C. Controlled Ventilation
76. Ans. — E. Severe Pyloric stenosis
77. Ans. — C. During controlled respiration
78. Ans. — E. All of the above
79. Ans. — D. Both A and B are true
80. Ans. — B. Thiopentone

    Thiopentone is a depressant of respiratory centre, depending on dose and rate of injection, antagonized by surgical stimuli and potentiated by opioids.
81. Ans. — D. Positive end pressure ventilation
82. Ans. — A. ↑ resistance in circuit
83. Ans. — B. Buprenorphine

84. Ans. — C. 6-7 L/mm
85. Ans. — A. Aspiration of gastric contents

    That is why adequate preparation (fasting) is necessary before giving GA.
86. Ans. — A. Scalenus anterior
87. Ans. — B. Hypotension
88. Ans. — A. A catalyst
89. Ans. — D. Skeletal muscle
90. Ans. — E. None of the above
91. Ans. — D. All of the above
92. Ans. — E. Both C and D are true
93. Ans. — B. Isoprenaline
94. Ans. — C. Overnight mechanical ventilation
95. Ans. — A. Transposition of the great arteries
96. Ans. — D. Hypothermia
97. Ans. — A. 25/8 mm Hg
98. Ans. — C. Elective overnight mechanical ventilation.
99. Ans. — C. Paraoxysmal supra-ventricular tachycardia.
100. Ans. — B. Esmolol

    Esmolol is a cardioselective beta one blocker having half life of less than 10 min and action lasts 15-20 min after terminating I.V. transfusion. It is used in AF, PSVT, HT and early MI.
101. Ans. — B. The left radial artery pulsations are absent.
102. Ans. — A. Ephedrine
103. Ans. — D. Cause bradycardia and a decrease in cardiac output.
104. Ans. — C. Botulinum toxin
105. Ans. — E. Beta-adrenergic blocking agents
106. Ans. — D. Due to stimulation of the Edinger Westphal nucleus.
107. Ans. — A. Platelets
108. Ans. — E. 233 mEq
109. Ans. — B. Jugular vein pressure
110. Ans. — A. 4 hours
111. Ans. — C. 1.0 to 1.5
112. Ans. — D. Dopamine
113. Ans. — B. Twice the viscosity of water
114. Ans. — C. Dipamine
115. Ans. — B. 7.7

116.	Ans. — C.	Nitroprusside
117.	Ans. — C.	Vomiting
118.	Ans. — D.	Both A and B are true
119.	Ans. — A.	Complete block
120.	Ans. — C.	At the same level as cricoid cartilage.
121.	Ans. — B.	Lateral to subclavian artery
122.	Ans. — C.	T4
123.	Ans. — B.	IX
124.	Ans. — B.	1.2-1.6 cms
125.	Ans. — B.	10 to 11 cm
126.	Ans. — B.	25°
127.	Ans. — D.	55°
128.	Ans. — C.	85%
129.	Ans. — A.	Remain normal or increase slightly
130.	Ans. — C.	7 : 1
131.	Ans. — B.	The arterioles
132.	Ans. — D.	The Cushing reflex raises arterial pressure.
133.	Ans. — D.	Myocardial O_2 demand
134.	Ans. — E.	The salivary glands
135.	Ans. — A.	Increase in mathaemoglobin
136.	Ans. — C.	Cyclophosphamide
137.	Ans. — D.	Dobutamine
138.	Ans. — D.	Ohio
139.	Ans. — B.	A hemolytic reaction
140.	Ans. — D.	Dilutional coagulopathy
141.	Ans. — A.	2% of blood volume
142.	Ans. — D.	2, 3 DPG
143.	Ans. — D.	Dextran
144.	Ans. — B.	CPD
145.	Ans. — C.	Beer-lambert's law
146.	Ans. — C.	Posterior 1/3rd
147.	Ans. — B.	Cuffed endotracheal tube
148.	Ans. — D.	Prone
149.	Ans. — A.	Potent anaesthesia action
150.	Ans. — C.	Injection of gallamine
151.	Ans. — A.	40
152.	Ans. — C.	23,000 feet
153.	Ans. — B.	Indicate flow rate of gases
154.	Ans. — A.	Aspirin
155.	Ans. — E.	Ethylene

156.	Ans. — D.	Toxic goitre
157.	Ans. — C.	Don't apply grease to valves repeatedly during storage.
158.	Ans. — B.	1.34
159.	Ans. — D.	A and B are correct
160.	Ans. — B.	Above which it will not liquify despite increased pressure.
161.	Ans. — A.	Diabetic alkalosis
162.	Ans. — D.	All of the above
163.	Ans. — B.	Carina
164.	Ans. — A.	Gas Cylinders
165.	Ans. — D.	A and B are true
166.	Ans. — C.	Hypoxemia
167.	Ans. — B.	Deep anaesthesia
168.	Ans. — C.	Decreases in Lactate/Pyruvate ratio in blood. It also causes fall in ICT and also ionized calcium in blood producing Respiratory alkalosis.
169.	Ans. — C.	Thiopentone
170.	Ans. — B.	Use cotton dresses
171.	Ans. — A.	Continuous flow type
172.	Ans. — D.	All of the above
173.	Ans. — A.	Most often causes transient hypertension
174.	Ans. — C.	Right to left shunts
175.	Ans. — B.	Deep anaesthesia
176.	Ans. — D.	Expiratory reserve volume
177.	Ans. — B.	Equal to minute volume. In this there is no rebreathing, if the fresh gas supply is more than 5 L/min in a 70 Kg patient.
178.	Ans. — C.	L3
179.	Ans. — B.	Elevation of head end of bed
180.	Ans. — E.	All of the above
181.	Ans. — C.	Rima Glottidis
182.	Ans. — B.	Functional Residual Capacity
183.	Ans. — E.	All of the above
184.	Ans. — A.	At rest the rate of O_2 uptake is decreased.
185.	Ans. — D.	Alveolar hypoventilation
186.	Ans. — D.	Histotoxic hypoxia
187.	Ans. — B.	Carbon Monoxide poisoning. The body is pinkish.

188. Ans. — A. To and Fro

189. Ans. — B. Few point hygrometre

190. Ans. — C. Tongue fall backwards and obstruct the posterior nasal opening.

191. Ans. — B. 3rd to 6th cervical vertebra

192. Ans. — B. S2 vertebra

193. Ans. — B. 31

194. Ans. — B. 58

195. Ans. — D. A + B

196. Ans. — A. 4 to 8 mesh

197. Ans. — A. Open system

198. Ans. — A. Mapelson A system

199. Ans. — B. Arterial PO_2

200. Ans. — D. All of the above

201. Ans. — B. 0.8

202. Ans. — B. Hypotonic food

203. Ans. — A. Tachycardia

Tachycardia and ventricular ectopi are important.

204. Ans. — B. 30-40

205. Ans. — A. Encapsulated receptors

206. Ans. — B. Lateral position

207. Ans. — A. Short operation with spontaneous breathing.

208. Ans. — A. Obstruction of air way

209. Ans. — A. It is excreted through kidneys

210. Ans. — C. Digitalis

Other methods used by sodium polystrene sulphate (Resonium-A) 30g in methyl-cellulose as enema, 20 ml of 10% Ca gluconate I/C, Peritoneal dialysis or Haemodialysis.

211. Ans. — D. 110-130c.c/square meter/minute

212. Ans. — C. Angiotensin

213. Ans. — D. All of the above

214. Ans. — D. All of the above

215. Ans. — B. Tall

216. Ans. — C. 0.5—1.0

217. Ans. — B. Pulse strength decreases

218. Ans. — A. 30% of tidal volume

219. Ans. — C. Decreased concentration of oxygenated haemoglobin.

220. Ans. — B. Ethylene

221. Ans. — C. 1/6th of total cardiac output

222. Ans. — B. 10 mm Hg

223. Ans. — A. Spinal cord

224. Ans. — C. Posterior horn cells

225. Ans. — C. Just below the vocal cord

226. Ans. — B. Flexion of neck with extension of atlanto-occipital joint.

227. Ans. — D. Minimum alveolar concentration

MAC (%) of ether is 1.9, of Halothane 0.75, Enflurane 1-68, Isoflurane 1.2, Desflurane 60, Sevoflurane 2.0, Nitrous oxide 105 Cyclopropane 9.2, Chloroform 0.8, TCE 0.2 and of Methoxyflurane 0.16.

228. Ans. — C. 60% of body weight

229. Ans. — A. 75 ml/kg of body weight

230. Ans. — D. Only A and B are true

231. Ans. — C. Electropexy

232. Ans. — D. Fat

233. Ans. — D. All of the above

234. Ans. — D. 10 days to 18 days

235. Ans. — C. 15% of estimated blood volume

236. Ans. — C. Compression of aorta and vena cava by the gravid uterus when lying supine.

237. Ans. — C. Induction and recovery

238. Ans. — D. All of the above

239. Ans. — A. First trimester

240. Ans. — B. Ischial tuberosity and greater trochanter

241. Ans. — D. Endotracheal intubation

Laryngeal complications of endotracheal intubation are ulceration, necrosis and stenosis.

242. Ans. — A. Lumbar 1st

243. Ans. — C. L1 2 3 4

244. Ans. — E. S2

245. Ans. — A. Hyper extention of head with elevation of jaw.

246. Ans. — C. I.P.P.V decreases the physiological dead space.

247. Ans. — D. PO2 of venous blood is 100 mm of mercury.

248. Ans. — D. Partial pressure of CO_2 in venous blood is 40 mm of mercury.

249.	Ans. — D.	Middle ear
250.	Ans. — B.	Adequate Analgesia
251.	Ans. — E.	Both B and C are true
252.	Ans. — A.	Left Ventricular failure
253.	Ans. — D.	All of the above
254.	Ans. — B.	Eisenmenger Syndrome
255.	Ans. — A.	Kety-Schmidt method
256.	Ans. — B.	Displacement of tube or obstruction

Surgical emphysema, haemorrhage and infection are common complications.

257. Ans. — B. Fall in respiratory rate

258. Ans. — A. Sympathomimetic drugs

259. Ans. — C. 85% Adrenaline and 15% of Noradrenaline.

260. Ans. — E. All of the above

261. Ans. — E. All of the above

262. Ans. — D. All of the above

263. Ans. — C. 50-80 mmol/day (mEQ/day)

264. Ans. — B. Urine

265. Ans. — B. Buffers

266. Ans. — B. Oncotic

267. Ans. — C. Overhydration

268. Ans. — E. All of the above

269. Ans. — A. Decreased concentration of plasma potassium.

270. Ans. — A. Decreased cardiac output

The chances of barotrauma are high and penumothorax, air embolism and pneumoperitoneum may result.

271. Ans. — D. Intravenous block

272. Ans. — B. 10 gm/dl

273. Ans. — D. No valves used

274. Ans. — B. Arterial blood

275. Ans. — B. Low molecular weight dextran

276. Ans. — A. 4—10 minutes

277. Ans. — D. Perforating injury of the eye

278. Ans. — C. Reduces regional arterial resistance in the kidney.

279. Ans. — D Central hypoventilation

280. Ans. — B. Atropine

281. Ans. — A. Decreased $PaCO_2$

282. Ans. — A. Organophosphorus poisoning

283. Ans. — A. Rapid Y descent

284. Ans. — B. Adrenaline

285. Ans. — C. Hypoglycemia

286. Ans. — A. Pneumothorax

287. Ans. — B. 5-10

288. Ans. — D. Posterior arytenoid paralysis

289. Ans. — B. 15-45%

290. Ans. — E. Cardiac arrhythmias

291. Ans. — B. Pancuronium

Sometimes, Pancuronium causes stimulation of myocardium and rise in pulse rate and B.P. and block vagal muscarinic receptors.

292. Ans. — D. Cyclopropane

293. Ans. — B. 0.04%

294. Ans. — B. Methyl isocyanide

295. Ans. — A. Increase dose of drug

296. Ans. — B. Constricts systemic vasculature

297. Ans. — B. 20

298. Ans. — B. 5 gm%

299. Ans. — D. 20%

300. Ans. — C. Urine output

301. Ans. B. 10 mm Hg

302. Ans. — C. 70%

303. Ans. — B. < 40 mm Hg < 70%

304. Ans. — C. 20 mg

305. Ans. — D. 30 mg

306. Ans. — B. Apex of orbit lateral to optic nerve.

307. Ans. — D. Main bronchus

308. Ans. — D. All of the above

309. Ans. — D. Eye opening, motor functions and best verbal response

310. Ans. — D. IV Tensilon

311. Ans. — A. Regenerating cholinesterase

312. Ans. — C. Reflex bronchospasm due to parasympathetic stress at a different site.

313. Ans. — D. O_2 intoxication

314. Ans. — E. All of the above

315. Ans. — E. High flow insufflation

316. Ans. — A. Respiratory acidosis

317. Ans. — D. 6 months
318. Ans. — B. Boiling
319. Ans. — B. 15-25 mm Hg
320. Ans. — D. Free nerve endings
321. Ans. — B. Obeying motor command
322. Ans. — B. Nor adrenaline
323. Ans. — B. 13-14
324. Ans. — C. 12-14 cm
325. Ans. — E. All of the above
326. Ans. — B. Facial nerve
327. Ans. — D. 1.0 mg
328. Ans. — C. Repeated ectopics
329. Ans. — B. d-tubocurare
330. Ans. — A. Aspiration pneumonia

Mendelson syndrome is common.

331. Ans. — A. Scalenus anticus
332. Ans. — B. 6 cm
333. Ans. — B. O_2 uptake/minute/kg
334. Ans. — C. Neck muscles
335. Ans. — C. 6
336. Ans. — B. 15
337. Ans. — C. 15 seconds
338. Ans. — C. Morphine

Special care is necessary on infants under 6 months aged, feeble and debilitated and patients with a raised intracranial pressure.

339. Ans. — D. Evaporation

It is used to localize the segments to be anaesthesised. pCO_2, suprarenal insufficiency, myasthenia, myotonia, hypothyroidism, asthma, raised ICT, respiratory depression, hepatic or renal failure, acute alcoholism, diverticulitis and labour. It kills by causing respiratory arrest.

340. Ans. — E. All of the above
341. Ans. — C. In 2 persons, CPR ratio is 5 : 1

About 12-20 times/min operator blows into victim's mouth about twice the amount of normal tidal volume.

342. Ans. — B. Lifting jaw forward
343. Ans. — C. Radial artery
344. Ans. — E. None of the above
345. Ans. — A. Monitoring of concentration of exhaled CO_2

346. Ans. — A. Massive pleural effusion
347. Ans. — E. All of the above
348. Ans. — D. Mitral regurgitation
349. Ans. — B. Trendelenburg position
350. Ans. — C. Mitral stenosis
351. Ans. — D. VSD
352. Ans. — D. Ayre's T piece
353. Ans. — C. Noisy breathing
354. Ans. — A. Inhalation
355. Ans. — B. Venti mask
356. Ans. — A. Provide airtight seal in trachea
357. Ans. — A. Diazepam
358. Ans. — C. 5% xylocaine with dextrose
359. Ans. — D. S2
360. Ans. — A. 16%
361. Ans. — A. Internal diameter of the tube in mm
362. Ans. — A. Halothane
363. Ans. — B. 100
364. Ans. — B. 1.5-2 inches

Chest is compressed upto 1-1.5 inches. It is given at a rate of 60/mt.

365. Ans. — A. Touch
366. Ans. — D. Taste
367. Ans. — C. 3.5%
368. Ans. — A. 100 ml
369. Ans. — C. Pralidoxine
370. Ans. — B. Should be as far as possible from the patients.
371. Ans. — D. Neck lift
372. Ans. — B. 1.5 times
373. Ans. — B. 2
374. Ans. — C. CO_2 and N_2O
375. Ans. — A. Miniature end plate potentials

The action is blocked by depolarising agents, non-depolarising agents and toxins.

376. Ans. — A. Between first and second lumbar spines.
377. Ans. — B. hypotension
378. Ans. — B. Joules-Thompson
379. Ans. — B. Sodium nitroprusside
380. Ans. — B. Respiratory rate 33/min
381. Ans. — B. Right venticular pressure
382. Ans. — B. Frozen erythrocytes

383. Ans. — C. Microthrombus in pulmonary vessels.

384. Ans. — D. Administration of I.V fluids

385. Ans. — B. Liver

386. Ans. — A. CVP

In hypovolemia, the systolic BP should if possible be restored to at least 100 mgHg (when the blood volume is probably not less than 70% of normal).

387. Ans. — B. 33%

388. Ans. — B. Equal to minute volume

389. Ans. — D. Hyderallazine cystathione synthetase

390. Ans. — D. ↓ ICT

391. Ans. — A. ↑ Bleeding

392. Ans. — B. Maintain airway

393. Ans. — B. Heimlich's manoeuvre

394. Ans. — D. Multicentric bronchogenic cyst

395. Ans. — B. Increased SA node activity

396. Ans. — A. Endotracheal intubation

397. Ans. — A. Paralysis of nerve supply from

398. Ans. — C. Tubercular cavity

399. Ans. — A. Respiratory stimulant

400. Ans. — D. ↑ Skin colour

401. Ans. — A. Molybdenum steel

Cylinders are made of molybdenum steel and checked for tensile strength, flattening, impact and bend tests and hydraulic or pressure test.

402. Ans. — A. 5 microns

Vaporizers, may be drawn over or machine gas driven plenum. Concentration distal to vaporizer depends on SVP (Saturated Vapour Pressure) of inhalation agent, temperature diverted to the vaporizing chambers. Surface area of vapour chamber including wick, flow characteristics and amount of liquid in vapour chamber.

403. Ans. — A. Equal

404. Ans. — A. Viscosity is proportional to shear stress.

405. Ans. — A. To assess airway patency

406. Ans. — C. 1, 2, 3 and 4

407. Ans. — A. Propofol

408. Ans. — C. CCF

Breathing air, 100 ml of plasma dissolves 0.3 ml oxygen. Breathing 100% oxygen at 1 atmosphere. 100 ml plasma will dissolve 2.1 ml oxygen whereas at 2 atmosphere, it will dissolve 4.2 ml oxygen.

409. Ans. — C. For easy intubation

410. Ans. — D. Treacher Collins syndrome

411. Ans. — A. Succinylcholine

412. Ans. — A. Pul. embolism

413. Ans. — B. Prolonged surgeries

414. Ans. — A. Needs to be decreased as they augment hypotension & muscle relaxation

415. Ans. — A. Intracardiac

416. Ans. — B. Endotracheal tube

417. Ans. — D. Nasal catheter

418. Ans. — C. Etomidate

419. Ans. — C. Venous air embolism

420. Ans. — B. Due to the lack of sitmulation by CO_2 anoxia can go into dangerous levels.

421. Ans. — C. Morphine

422. Ans. — D. Prevents barotrauma

423. Ans. — A. Their general condition

424. Ans. — C. 93 ±10

425. Ans. — C. Increased risk of gastric regurgitation

426. Ans. — D. Intramuscular

427. Ans. — C. Crystalloid infusion

428. Ans. — D. Hypoventilation

429. Ans. — B. 150 ml

430. Ans. — A. Hypothermia

431. Ans. — C. End tidal CO_2

432. Ans. — A. Pin index

433. Ans. — B. It decreases turbulance

Helium was isolated by Sir W. Ramsey (1852-1916) in 1895. It is inert, colourless odourless gas with Mol. Wt. - 4 boiling point - 26.9°C. It is second lightest gas (to hydrogen). A mixture of 21% oxygen and 79% helium has a SG of 341. It is also used to measure lung volumes and like nitrogen, prevents lung collapse.

434. Ans. — B. Carbon monoxide

Early and Rapid removal of CO from body is done by good ventilation, IPPV if necessary 85% of CO is in Hemoglobin and 15% in myoglobin. Oxygen is the primary therapy. Brain damage is both time and dose related. Oxygen therapy reduces half life of CO to less than 30 min, restores phosphocreatinine and ATP production, restores glucose utilization, reduces succinate levels to normal and reduces lactate/pyruvate ratio. Blood samples are taken for HbCO. The absorption spectrum peaks at 590-610 nM. Poor prognosis is indicated by delay in treatment (of over 2h), age over 40 years, metabolic acidosis, coma, cardiac ischemia and cerebral abnormalities on CT scan.

435. Ans. — D. 15 : 2

436. Ans. — C. Hudson's mask

437. Ans. — C. He wanted to see if there was an oculocardiac reflex.

438. Ans. — D. 30-50 L/min.

439. Ans. — A. Black cylinder with white shoulders

440. Ans. — B. Induction with intravenous propofol and N_2O and oxygen for maintenance.

* In case of Duchenne's muscular dystrophy the most appropriate anaesthetic agent of choice is Propofol and N_2O and oxygen for maintenance

* In hepatic failure anaesthetic agent of choice is - isofluorane.

* In renal failure, Raised ICT anaesthetic of choice is - Isofluorane.

Anaesthesia Gas Delivery System :

a) Spontaneous Breathing - Maplesen A or Magill system, flow rate of gas is 5 lit/min.

b) In iPPV - (1) Maplesen D or Bain Coaxial System (for child and adults)

c) Maplesen E or Ayre's T tube, for infant & young children, Flow rate = 2 x 5 L. (Min volume).

441. Ans. — A. Maplesen A

442. Ans. — A. Fat embolism

Fat Embolism :

* MC form of non-thrombotic embolism which usually follows:

a) Severe road accident injury

b) Fractures around great veins.

* Earliest sign - Fat emboli in retinal vessels, striate haemorrhage fluffy patches of exudates on Retina.

* T/t - oxygenation, heparinization, I/v LMW Dextran.

443. Ans. — C. Systemic toxicity of local anaesthetics.

444. Ans. — C. Caudal anaesthesia

* Regional anaesthesia is the technique of choice for elective caesarean section.

Techniques are : - Spinal anaesthesia
- Epidural anaesthesia
- Combined spinal Epidural anaesthesia

The proportion of Mothers being delivered under general anaesthesia by Caesarean section depends on many factors. It is gradually alling.

* The primary advantages of GA for Caesariean section is the reliability and rapidity of onset of astate in which the operation is performed.

* Caudal anaesthesia is unpopular because of the risk of introducing needle passing through the mother's sacrum and rectum and into fetal presenting parts.

445. Ans. — A. Sevoflurane

"Intracranial pressure increased at high inspired concentrations of sevoflurane but this effect is minimal over the 0.5-1.0 MAC range."

446. Ans. — A. Jackson Rees' modificatin of Ayres' T Piece.

- Ayre's T piece is an example of maplesen E.

- It is advocated primarily for use in infants and young children.

- Jackson Ree's modified it and added a bag for monitoring and IPPV. (Maplesen F)

- Gases can be scavenged.

- The main advantage of the T-piece technique is the absence of resistance to expiration, a factor of crucial importance in small children.

- Efficacy of systems with spontaneous respiration.

A > D & E > C > B

Although, A is more efficaceous but E is more suitable for infants.

447.   Ans. — D.   Assist - control ventilation (ACV)

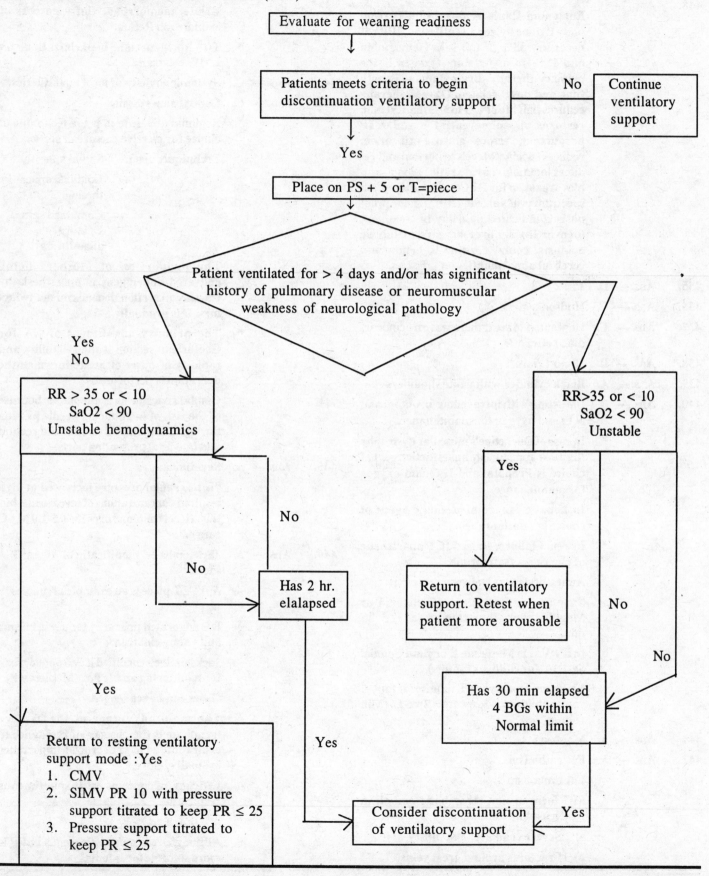

448.   Ans. — D.   In a patient with a large tumor in the oral cavity.

* Reports support the use of the LMA for difficult airway management during cardiopulmonary resuscitation.

* Difficult intubation

- Insertion of LMA or combitube

* LMA have little effect on intra-ocular pressure. Therefore, they may be useful for airway management of patients undergoing examination of the eye under anaesthesia. The absence of face mask may facilitate the examination.

LMA has been used for extra-ocular and intra-ocular surgery including retinopathy surgery in ex-premature infants. (better access the surgical field and does not affects the IOT).

449.   Ans. — B.   Classifies the Bain system as maples on D.

450.   Ans. — C.   33 degrees C

REVIEW PAPER-I

(Based on Difficult & Important MCQ's)

1. The optimum temperature for heating ammonium nitrate to produce nitrous oxide is ——— ° C.
   A. 150
   B. 250
   C. 350
   D. 400

2. An active scavenging gas system should be able to tolerate constant flows of ——— L/min with peak gas flows of ——— L/min respectively.
   A. 50, 110
   B. 75, 130
   C. 110, 180
   D. 110, 230

3. Tissue oxygen requirement in a neonate is ——— ml/kg/min.
   A. 2
   B. 4
   C. 6
   D. 12

4. In Tracheostomy, tube cuff pressure should be maintained ——— mm Hg.
   A. Below 20
   B. 20-25
   C. 25-30
   D. 30-40

5. Air embolism may be diagnosed using following except :
   A. Pre-cordial auscultation to detect a mill-wheel murmur.
   B. Capnography where a sudden rise in end expiratory CO_2 is seen.
   C. A pulmonary artery catheter.
   D. A doppler ultrasound in the presence of as little as 0.5 ml of intravascular air.

6. Autologous transfusion is possible with a predonation of upto ——— units.
   A. 4
   B. 6
   C. 10
   D. 12

7. Blood salvage technique is especially useful in patients undergoing ——— surgery.
   A. Neuro
   B. Dermato
   C. Cardiac
   D. Gastro

8. Preoperative seizure commonly occurs due to :
   A. Low K+
   B. Low Na+
   C. High Mg++
   D. Hypothermia

9. Activated clotting time is approximately ——— sec.
   A. 5
   B. 50
   C. 100
   D. 200

10. Following is contraindicated in a patient with malignant hyperpyrexia :
    A. Propofol
    B. Isoflurane
    C. Halothane
    D. None of the above

11. Recognized complications of hypotensive anaesthesia are the following except :
    A. Retraction ischemia
    B. Blindness
    C. Splenic infarction
    D. ↑ incidence of DVT

12. The following will prolong the duration of action of suxamethonium except :
    A. Ecothiopate
    B. Isoflurane
    C. Cyclophosphamide
    D. Neostigmine

13. When anaesthetizing patients with asthma, the following phase should be prolonged :
    A. Inspiratory
    B. Expiratory
    C. Both
    D. None

14. Following may exacerbate the weakness of well controlled myasthemia gravis except :
    A. Hypokalemia
    B. Ciprofloxacin
    C. Edrophanium
    D. Doxycycline

15. Following may be omitted from inspired gas mixture of a patient undergoing laser surgery to upper pathway :
    A. Nitrogen
    B. Helium
    C. Isoflurane
    D. None of the above

16. In hypotensive anaesthesia, failure of cerebral auto regulation occurs if mean arterial B.P. (MABP) is below ——— mm Hg.
    A. 50
    B. 60
    C. 70
    D. 80

Ans.	1. B	2. B	3. C	4. B	5. B	6. B	7. C	8. B	9. C	10. B
	11. C	12. B	13. B	14. D	15. D	16. A				

17. In hypotensive anaesthesia, GFR is reduced if Mean arterial B.P is below —— mm Hg.
   - A. 60
   - B. 70
   - C. 80
   - D. 90

18. Nitrous oxide is —— times more suluble in blood than nitrogen.
   - A. 20
   - B. 24
   - C. 34
   - D. 44

19. Glycine solution used for transurethral resection of prostate is absorbed at a rate of approximately —— ml/min.
   - A. 5
   - B. 10
   - C. 20
   - D. 40

20. Pulmonary oedema may result if the usual lymphatic drainage of —— ml per day is exceeded.
   - A. 100
   - B. 250
   - C. 500
   - D. 750

21. Hypothermia results in a decrease in MAC requirement of ——% per degree of temperature fall.
   - A. 3
   - B. 7
   - C. 15
   - D. 25

22. In hypothermia, there is decline in level of consciousness below ——°C.
   - A. 32
   - B. 30
   - C. 28
   - D. 20

23. The filter found in blood giving sets have pore size usually between —— mm.
   - A. 10-20
   - B. 50-120
   - C. 180-200
   - D. 210-240

24. The following are suggestive of an air embolism in and at risk patient except :
   - A. Coughing
   - B. Bradycardia
   - C. Hypotension
   - D. Jugular venous distension

25. The following may exacerbate the symptoms of multiple sclerosis :
   - A. Cold
   - B. Exercise
   - C. GA
   - D. Regional anaesthesia

26. 'Coronary steal' is typically seen with :
   - A. Sevoflurane
   - B. Desflurane
   - C. Isoflurane
   - D. Enflurane

27. A substance flowing through a tube is attracted to its walls. This is —— effect.
   - A. Bernouli
   - B. Laplace
   - C. Coanda
   - D. Dalton

28. Total pressure exerted by a gas mixture is sum of the individual partial pressures of its constituents. This is ——law.
   - A. Grahem
   - B. Charles
   - C. Avagadro
   - D. Dalton

29. The dural sac ends at :
   - A. T-12
   - B. L-2
   - C. LO_4
   - D. S-2

30. Etheringlon Wilson technique is used for:
   - A. Subarachnoid anaesthesia
   - B. Extradural block
   - C. Intradural block
   - D. Cardiac resuscitation

31. Gattinoni method is used for extracorpeal removal of:
   - A. Blood
   - B. Urine
   - C. CO_2
   - D. CSF

32. Guitierrez's sign is most useful in extradural analgesia in:
   - A. Thorax
   - B. Abdomen
   - C. Pelvis
   - D. Extremity

33. Durran's sign is that in a an unconscious patient the rapid injection of liquid into the —— space is accompanied by the—— in rate and depth of respiration.
   - A. Extradural, increase
   - B. Extradural, decrease
   - C. Intradural, decrease
   - D. Intradural, increase

34. Wake up test is used in operations for:
   - A. Cervical sponylosis
   - B. Kyphoscoliosis
   - C. Hydrocephalus
   - D. Buerger's disease

35. Critical velocity of flow is calculated by:
   - A. $\dfrac{(2000 \times \text{Viscosity})}{(\text{diameter} \times \text{density})}$
   - B. $\dfrac{2000 \times \text{density}^2}{(\text{diameter} \times \text{viscosity})}$
   - C. $\dfrac{(2000 \times \text{viscosity}^2}{(\text{diameter} \times \text{density})}$
   - D. $\dfrac{(2000 \times \text{diameter}^4)}{(\text{density} \times \text{viscosity})}$

36. Air embolism is specially dangerous in the following except:
   - A. ASD
   - B. AS
   - C. PDA
   - D. VSD

Ans.	17. A	18. C	19. C	20. C	21. B	22. B	23. C	24. B	25. B	26. C
	27. C	28. D	29. D	30. C	31. C	32. A	33. A	34. B	35. A	36. B

37. Critical flow rate is related to
   A. Square of density
   B. Reynold's number
   C. Temperature of fluid
   D. pH of fluid

38. Following are true about atmospheric pressure at sea level except:
   A. 161.33k pa
   B. 1.0133×105 N/m²
   C. 14.7 lb/in²
   D. 10350 cm H_2O

39. Classic ECG changes of hyperkalemia occurs when its plasma concentration is usually above —— mmol/L.
   A. 4.0
   B. 4.5
   C. 5.5
   D. 6.5

40. Difficult endotracheal intubation may be anticipated in :
   A. Shy-Drager syndrome
   B. Pierre-Robin syndrome
   C. Klippel-Feil syndrome
   D. Treachre-Collins syndrome

41. The following can occur after dextran infusion :
   A. Decreased coagubility
   B. Rouleaux formation
   C. Renal tubular damage
   D. None of the above

42. Cross matching may be difficult when —— is infused :
   A. Dextran - 40
   B. Dextran - 70
   C. Both
   D. None of the above

43. Saturated vapour pressure (mmHg at 20°C) of following is minimum :
   A. Diethyl ether
   B. Halothane
   C. Methoxyflurane
   D. TCE

44. Saturated vapour pressure (mmHg at 20°C) of following is maximum :
   A. Isoflurane
   B. Halothane
   C. Enflurane
   D. Diethyl ether

45. Which of the following Mepelson system does not have any clinical role :
   A. A
   B. B
   C. C
   D. E

46. Parry Brown position is used for surgery in :
   A. Head
   B. Thorax
   C. Abdomen
   D. Pelvis

47. Term 'Pendelluft' refers to :
   A. Level of consciousness
   B. Type of breathing
   C. Controlled body temperature
   D. Fluid loss in surgery

48. 'Pop-off' valve is a :
   A. Expiratory valve
   B. Inspiratory valve
   C. Artificial heart valve
   D. Artificial shunt

49. Following are true about propofol except :
   A. Lipid soluble
   B. High incidence of anaphylaxis
   C. Induction within 10-30 sec after I.V.
   D. Apnea less common than thiopentone

50. Dose of Etomidate is —— mg/kg I.V.
   A. 0.3
   B. 1.0
   C. 1.2
   D. 2.4

51. All of the following are features of protein-C except :
   A. Vitamin K-dependent
   B. Proteolytic enzyme
   C. Inhibited by Heparin
   D. Exerts its effects by Factors V and VIII degradation

52. Hysteresis is best seen in :
   A. Kidneys
   B. Lungs
   C. Brain
   D. Testis

53. Rees modification of Ayre's T-piece is classified as Mepelsen —— system.
   A. D
   B. E
   C. F
   D. G

54. Ropivacaine is chemically similar to :
   A. Prilocaine
   B. Bupivacaine
   C. Etidocaine
   D. Mepivacaine

55. Dose of Propofol in elderly is —— mg/kg.
   A. 0.50
   B. 1.25
   C. 2.5
   D. 5.0

56. Characteristics of uncompensated metabolic acidosis are all except :
   A. Normal Pa CO_2
   B. Low pH
   C. Low bicarbonate
   D. None of the above

57. Loss of weight with normal or increased appetite may be found in following except :
   A. Thyrotoxicosis
   B. Diabetes mellitus
   C. Carcinoma stomach
   D. None of the above

58. Most potent vasodilator among the following is :
   A. Halothane
   B. Enflurane
   C. Sevoflurane
   D. Desflurane

59. Which of the following is not stable with Sodalime :
   A. Enflurane
   B. Isoflurane
   C. Sevoflurane
   D. Desflurane

Ans.	37. B	38. A	39. C	40. A	41. D	42. B	43. C	44. D	45. B	46. B
	47. B	48. A	49. D	50. A	51. C	52. B	53. C	54. B	55. B	56. D
	57. C	58. C	59. C							

60. Which of the following has lowest blood gas solubility :
    A. Enflurane
    B. Isoflurane
    C. Sevoflurane
    D. Desflurane

61. Which among the following is most resistant to 'Halothane hepatitis :
    A. Obese men
    B. Obese women
    C. Children
    D. Eldery

62. In 1951, Halothane was synthesized by :
    A. Ralph Waters
    B. Robert Macintosh
    C. Suckling
    D. Magill

63. According to Laplace's law, surface tension in the wall of a sphere is equal to :
    A. PR x 1.5
    B. PR x 4
    C. $\dfrac{PR \times 2}{4}$
    D. $\sqrt{P^2 R}$

64. Carbon dioxide was isolated by :
    A. Edmund Boyle
    B. Joseph Black
    C. Humphery Davy
    D. Griffith and Johnson

65. Following are present in Moffatt's solution except :
    A. Cocaine
    B. Ligocaine
    C. NaHCO3
    D. Adrenaline

66. Following drug may cause jaundice :
    A. Cimetidine
    B. Ranitidine
    C. Metronidazole
    D. All of the above

67. Baclofen is a derivative of :
    A. Dopamine
    B. GABA
    C. Glycine
    D. Tryptophan

68. 'Te-Ch' is a term used in :
    A. Alzheimer's disease
    B. Induced hypothermia
    C. Acupuncture
    D. Hypercarbia

69. 'Vascular waterfall' is dependent on the following except :
    A. Upstream pressure
    B. Pressure in the box
    C. Venous pressure
    D. None of the above

70. Ketamine was introduced as anaesthetic agent in :
    A. 1961
    B. 1963
    C. 1965
    D. 1967

71. If a patient with incapacitating systemic disease that is a constant threat to life is classified on ASA Physical Status Scale in class :
    A. II
    B. III
    C. IV
    D. V

72. 'Fast alveolus' has :
    A. High compliance low resistance
    B. Low compliance low resistance
    C. Low compliance high resistance
    D. High compliance high resistance

73. Bohr Enghoff equation is used calculate :
    A. $PaCO_2$
    B. Oxygen carrying capacity
    C. Physiological dead space
    D. Maximum lung capacity

74. Coanda Effect describes a phenomenon whereby —— flow through a tube with the Venturis tends to cling either to one side of the tube or to the other :
    A. Water
    B. Blood
    C. Gas
    D. Any of the above

75. Coplan's tube is used in :
    A. Bronchoscopy
    B. Microlaryngoscopy
    C. Endoscopy
    D. I/V alimentation

76. 'Dew' point is used to calculate :
    A. Viscosity
    B. Humidity
    C. Temperature
    D. Velocity

77. In 'space rescue' blanket, the metal used is :
    A. Lead
    B. Aluminium
    C. Chromium
    D. Bronze

78. Following are correct about sufentanil except :
    A. 600-700 times more potent than morphine
    B. Lipid soluble
    C. Dose is 5-10 mg in those breathing spontaneously
    D. Low therapeutic index

79. Among the following, which is longest acting :
    A. Subrachnoid morphine
    B. Extradural morphine
    C. Extradural diamorphine
    D. Extradural Methadone

80. Main side effect of Meptazinol is :
    A. Nausea and vomiting
    B. Convulsions
    C. Hypotension
    D. Cardiac arrthymias

81. 'TURP' syndrome is due to :
    A. Hypotension
    B. Hypothermia
    C. Hypoosmolarity
    D. Hypoxaemia

82. Which of the following is derived from alkaloid 'Toxiferin' :
    A. Vecuronium
    B. Alcuronium
    C. Atracuronium
    D. Pipecuronium

83. Which of the following drug cause vagal blockade as well as sympathomimetic action :
    A. Alcuronium
    B. Vecuronium
    C. Atracuronium
    D. Pancuronium

84. Histamine release is maximum with which non-depolarising drug :
    A. d-TC
    B. Gallamine
    C. Alcuronium
    D. Atracuronium

Ans.	60. D	61. C	62. C	63. C	64. B	65. B	66. A	67. B	68. C	69. C
	70. C	71. C	72. B	73. C	74. C	75. B	76. B	77. B	78. D	79. A
	80. A	81. C	82. B	83. D	84. A					

85. The name of von Recklinghausen is also associated with a :
    A. Vaporiser
    B. Cardiac valve
    C. Face mask
    D. Oscillotonometer

86. Waters' system (or to and fro system) comprises a Mepelsen —— breathing system :
    A. A
    B. C
    C. D
    D. E

87. Weaver's syndrome is characterized by :
    A. Adrenal failure
    B. Craniofacial deformities
    C. Diabetes mellitus
    D. Constrictive pericarditis

88. Ritey's and Filley's equations are used to calculate :
    A. PACO2
    B. PAO2
    C. PECO2
    D. None of the above

89. Slow alveoli have :
    A. High compliance, high resistance
    B. High compliance, low resistance
    C. Low compliance, low resistance
    D. Low compliance, high resistance

90. The best way to correct continuous 'Fighting the ventilator is :
    A. Correct ventilator
    B. Give Oxygen
    C. Give CO$_2$
    D. Remove ventilator

91. 'Gelofusine's is :
    A. Antihypertensive
    B. Coagulant
    C. Volume expander
    D. Antitussive

92. Moffatt's solution is best used in surgery of :
    A. Nose
    B. Heart
    C. Brain
    D. Liver

93. Torricellian vacuum is the working principle of :
    A. Entonox
    B. Mercury barometer
    C. Bernouilli nebulizer
    D. Depot Insulin injection

94. Enoximone causes all of the following except :
    A. ↑ stroke volume
    B. Inotropic state
    C. ↑ cardiac output
    D. ↑ afterloa

95. Pseudomembranous colitis is caused by all of the following except :
    A. Gentamycin
    B. Imipenam
    C. Metronidazole
    D. Clindamycin

96. Shoulder of Helium cylinder is.
    A. Brown/White
    B. Brown
    C. Grey
    D. Grey/White

97. 1 cm of H$_2$O is equivalent to —— mm Hg :
    A. 1.32
    B. 1.33
    C. 1.36
    D. 1.39

98. A bag of blood after 3 weeks storage contains —— ml of citrate phosphate.
    A. 53
    B. 57
    C. 63
    D. 67

99. Following is not true about composition of a bag of blood after 3 weeks storage :
    A. Plasma lactate 179 mmol/l
    B. Factors V and VII below 20%
    C. HCO$_3$- 11mmol/L
    D. Active platelets 5%

100. Oxygen flux is measured by :
    A. $\dfrac{Q \times SaO_2 \times Hb \times 10}{1.39}$

    B. $\dfrac{Q \times SaO_2 \times Hb \times 1.39}{10}$

    C. $\dfrac{Q \times (SaO_2 - SaCO_2) \times Hb}{10}$

    D. $\dfrac{Q \times (SaO_2 - SaCO_2) \times Hb \times 10}{1.39}$

101. The gastroesophageal junction may be made incompetent by :
    A. Deep Anaesthesia
    B. ↑ Intra-abdominal pressure
    C. Scleroderma
    D. Nasogastric sump tube

102. Which of the following is most important lead in detecting dysrhythmia during anaesthesia :
    A. I
    B. II
    C. III
    D. aVL

103. Tachycardia is persistent heart beat/min above :
    A. 72
    B. 80
    C. 90
    D. 100

104. On opening full mouth, soft palate, fauces and uvula are seen, it is classified as class—— (given by Mallampati) of laryngeal anatomy.
    A. 1
    B. 2
    C. 3
    D. 4

105. Lung resection is contraindicated in a patient whose FEV$_1$ is below—— litre :
    A. 0.8
    B. 1.0
    C. 1.2
    D. 2.2

106. On ECG, J-waves are seen in :
    A. Hypermagnesemia
    B. Wilson's disease
    C. Hypothermia
    D. Neuroleptic malignant syndrome

Ans.	85. D	86. B	87. A	88. A	89. A	90. D	91. C	92. A	93. B	94. D
	95. C	96. B	97. C	98. C	99. D	100. B	101. A,D	102. B	103. D	104. B
	105. A	106. C								

107. Cormack and Lehane score is used for :
    A. Dysrhythmia during anaesthesia
    B. BP variation in anaesthesia
    C. Difficult intubation
    D. Peadiatric trauma

108. For acute physiology and chronic health evaluation, following is used :
    A. ISS
    B. Mallampatti score
    C. APACHE
    D. Goldman index

109. According to National Institute for occupational safety and Health, N_2O concentration in the operating room should not exceed —— ppm.
    A. 10
    B. 15
    C. 25
    D. 50

110. The 'usual' leakage of fluid from pulmonary capillaries with lymphatics returning the fluid to the intravascular space is ——— ml/d.
    A. 50
    B. 100
    C. 250
    D. 500

111. Cardiff aldasorder is used to absorb :
    A. CO
    B. Halothane
    C. Cyclopropane
    D. Cyanide

112. The closing capacity of lung :
    A. Is same as closing volume
    B. Is closing volume plus residual volume
    C. Is closing volume minus residual volume
    D. Is tidal volume plus closing volume

113. Water has a specific heat of —— cal/g.
    A. 1
    B. 2
    C. 3
    D. 5

114. Absolute contraindication to lumbar epidural anaesthesia is :
    A. Bleeding diathesis with INR below 0.5
    B. History of polio
    C. Previous laminectomy at L5 level
    D. Abruption placenta

115. True about flumazenil is :
    A. 70% protein bound
    B. Plasma elimination half life is about 6 hours
    C. It also antagonises the effects of alcohol
    D. Accelerates recovery from halothane anaesthesia

116. True about the metabolism of atracurium is all except :
    A. Hypothermia inhibits
    B. Falling pH inhibits
    C. Eliminated by Hoffmann elimination
    D. None of the above

117. The maximum absorption of CO_2 by soda-lime is :
    A. 6
    B. 12
    C. 18
    D. 26

118. The minimum alveolar concentration of halothane is reduced by following except :
    A. Methyldopa
    B. Clonidine
    C. Ephedrine
    D. Reserpine

119. Following are used to measure the concentration of a gas or vapour except :
    A. Light emission
    B. Light absorption
    C. Thermal conductivity
    D. Refractive index
    E. None of the above

120. Polygeline, a urea linked gelatin solution is presented as —— % solution .
    A. 1
    B. 2.5
    C. 5
    D. 7.5

121. Which of the following is a skeletal muscle relaxant:
    A. Lithium
    B. Diltiazem
    C. Dantrolene
    D. None of the above

122. Prolonged action of non-depolarising neuromuscular blocking agents may be associated with :
    A. Hypermagnesemia
    B. Hypocalcemia
    C. Respiratory acidosis
    D. Metabolic alkalosis

123. In anaesthetic gas scavenging, nitrous oxide concentration and the level of halogenated agents should be below —— parts per million respectively.
    A. 50, 4
    B. 50, 2
    C. 25, 2
    D. 10, 1

124. In hypotensive anaesthesia, cerebral vasoconstricting effect of hypocarbia if mean arterial B.P. (MABP) is below —— mm Hg.
    A. 35
    B. 50
    C. 60
    D. 70

125. Malignant hyperpyrexia has its gene locus on the long arm of chromosome :
    A. 13
    B. 15
    C. 17
    D. 19

126. The following are likely sequelae after a near-drowning except :
    A. Cerebral oedema
    B. Profound acidosis
    C. Renal failure
    D. Acute pancreatitis

Ans.	107. C	108. C	109. C	110. D	111. B	112. C	113. A	114. D	115. C	116. C
	117. D	118. C	119. E	120. B	121. C	122. ALL	123. C	124. A	125. D	126. D

127. **Expiratory pause of a neonate is —— sec.**
   A. 0
   B. 5
   C. 1
   D. 2

128. **In acute attack of malignant hyperpyrexia the body temperature classically rise by ——°C per hour.**
   A. 0.5
   B. 1
   C. 2
   D. 3

129. **Myasthenia gravis may be associated with the following except :**
   A. Conn's syndrome
   B. Thyrotoxicosis
   C. Pernicious anaemia
   D. Rheumatoid arthritis

130. **Thiopentone is usually stored with —— % anhydrous sodium carbonate.**
   A. 2.5
   B. 4
   C. 6
   D. 7.5

131. **In retrobulbar block, —— ml of —— % lignocaine is commonly used.**
   A. 0.5, 1.0
   B. 1.0, 2.0
   C. 2.0, 2.0
   D. 5.0, 4.0

132. **The following may raise intraocular pressure :**
   A. IV lignocaine
   B. Beta blockers
   C. Ecthiopate
   D. Hypercarbia

133. **Gas flow is likely to be turbulent :**
   A. Below a Reynolds number of 500
   B. Above a Reynolds number of 1000
   C. Above a Reynolds number of 1500
   D. Above a Reynolds number of 2000

134. **Symptoms of air embolism are produced if air enters a vessel atleast at a rate of —— ml/kg/min.**
   A. 0.1
   B. 0.5
   C. 1.0
   D. 2.0

135. **The storage of blood with citrate, phosphate and dextrose provides a shelf life of —— days.**
   A. 15
   B. 21
   C. 30
   D. 45

136. **Sodium chloride, adenine, glucose and mannitol provides a shelf life of —— days.**
   A. 15
   B. 30
   C. 45
   D. 60

137. **At doses above 1000 ml/70 kg, hydroxyethyl starch decreases factor :**
   A. V
   B. VIII
   C. IX
   D. X

138. **The lumen of a Robertshaw tube is —— shaped.**
   A. B
   B. D
   C. M
   D. N

139. **Tare weight is the weight of cylinder when :**
   A. Full
   B. Empty
   C. Half-filled
   D. Any of the above

140. **Vaughan-Williams classification is used to classify :**
   A. Antihypertensives
   B. Antiarrythmic
   C. Antidiarhoeal
   D. Antimalarial

141. **Only —— % of manufactured oxygen is for medical use.**
   A. 1
   B. 10
   C. 20
   D. 40

142. **Boiling point of Enflurane is :**
   A. 49
   B. 50
   C. 56
   D. 64

143. **Swollen, cherry red epiglottis is seen in :**
   A. Laryngotracheitis
   B. Epiglottitis
   C. Diphtheria
   D. All of the above

144. **Hemoglobin is usually least at :**
   A. Birth
   B. 3 months
   C. 1 year
   D. 12 years

145. **Transfused RBC's have about —— % of normal 2, 3 DPG level.**
   A. 30
   B. 50
   C. 70
   D. 90

146. **One unit of blood (500 ml) is collected in a bag containing —— ml of citrate phosphate and Dextrose.**
   A. 30
   B. 50
   C. 70
   D. 110

147. **Critical pressure of carbon dioxide is ——bar.**
   A. 46.2
   B. 63.7
   C. 73.8
   D. 87.2

148. **Drugs to be avoided in epileptic patients are all except :**
   A. Propofol
   B. Etomidate
   C. Enflurane
   D. Isoflurane

149. **Spinal anaesthesia was introduced by :**
   A. Claude Bernard
   B. McKeeson
   C. Bier
   D. Ralph Watters

150. **Local analgesic properties of cocaine were first reported by :**
   A. Edmund Boyle
   B. Quincle
   C. Koller
   D. Freud

Ans.	127. A	128. C	129. A	130. C	131. C	132. D	133. C	134. B	135. B	136. C
	137. B	138. B	139. B	140. B	141. A	142. C	143. B	144. B	145. C	146. C
	147. C	148. D	149. C	150. C						

COMBINED MEDICAL SERVICES EXAMINATION
(Conducted by UPSC)

- It contains original solved papers from **1983 onwards**

- All papers are **Subjectwise & Yearwise** arranged

- Answers are given at the foot and **detailed explanations** are given at the end.

- Detailed **instructions** about this examination are given

- Important **references** to be read are also given

- Each year's paper is classified into two separate parts arranged subjectwise

- Book is suited for Quick revision before the examination and also to know its pattern

- High chance of repetition in this exam as well as in other UPSC conducted Exams

- Read the papers before undertaking preparation (to know the pattern), then read text and again check your knowledge by doing papers

- Also useful for **Civil Services Examination, Part I** (Medical Sciences) as the question Bank is same

- Also read book on **Civil Services Examination, Part I (Medical Sciences)** (by same author and publishers) as the **Question Bank** of two exams may overlap.

- All suggestions and Contributions are welcome and write to the Editor :
  Dr. M.S. Bhatia, D-1, Naraina Vihar, New Delhi-110028

CBS Publishers & Distributors Pvt. Ltd.
NEW DELHI • BANGALORE • PUNE • CHENNAI • COCHIN

REVIEW PAPER-II

(Based on Difficult & Important MCQ's)

1. The blood-brain barrier is not readily crossed by :
   A. Oxygen
   B. Potassium
   C Carbon dioxide
   D. Bicarbonate

2. Consciousness will first be lost by the unacclimated person when breathing air at an altitude of :
   A. 10,000 feet
   B. 18,000 feet
   C. 20,000 feet
   D. 35,000 feet

3. The "mass reflex" in a quadriplegic cause following except :
   A. Bladder and rectum evacuation
   B. Blood pressure swings
   C. Flexor-extensor motor spasms
   D. None of the above

4. Uremic patients have numerous pathophysiologic changes that may affect anaesthetic management. These include following except :
   A. Immunologic suppression
   B. Delayed gastric emptying
   C. Autonomic neuropathies
   D. Coagulopathies due primarily to deflicts in platelet count

5. In which pulmonary function test is Boyle's law used for the calculations :
   A. The single-breath CO test
   B. The N_2 washout test
   C. The O_2 diffusion test
   D. Body plethysmography

6. How much of a drop in pressure is required to obtain an air flow rate of 1/L/sec during normal inspiration:
   A. 1 cm H_2O
   B. 2 cm H_2O
   C. 3 cm H_2O
   D. 4 cm H_2O

7. The partial pressure of water vapor in saturated air at normal body temperature is :
   A. 10 mm Hg
   B. 20 mm Hg
   C. 35 mm Hg
   D. 47 mm Hg

8. In recent European literature, the SI (Systeme International d'Unites) units are used. In this system one kilopascal equals :
   A. 2.5 mm Hg
   B. 5.0 mm Hg
   C. 6.0 mm Hg
   D. 7.5 mm Hg

9. If the pressure is constant and 400 mL of water (viscosity = 1.0) flows through a tube in 30 seconds, how many milliliters of castor oil (viscosity = 9.9) will flow through the same tube in the same time:
   A. 300
   B. 200
   C. 90
   D. 40

10. An E cylinder of oxygen with a pressure reading of 1,600 psi will last approximately how many hours at a flow rate of 4 L/min:
    A. 1.50
    B. 1.75
    C. 2.00
    D. 2.25

11. Which of the following gases has (have paramagnetic properties that are utilized clinically in its (their) measurement:
    A. CO_2
    B. Nitrogen
    C. Cyclopropane
    D. Oxygen

12. Infrared analysis may be used for the determination of following except :
    A. Carbon dioxide
    B. Nitrous oxide
    C. Carbon monoxide
    D. Oxygen

13. In the commonly used temperature scales, + 273 K (Kelvin) equals :
    A. 212°F
    B. 0°C
    C. 100°C
    D. 32°F

14. In calculating the uptake of halothane, consideration must be given to the :
    A. Second gas effect
    B. Concentration effect
    C. Loss of anaesthetic agent to the soda lime
    D. All of the above

Ans.	1. D	2. C	3. D	4. D	5. D	6. B	7. D	8. D	9. D	10. C
	11. D	12. D	13. B	14. D						

15. **Concerning nitrous oxide and oxygen stored in standard E cylinders :**
    A. Both exist in a liquid state in a full cylinder.
    B. The same volume of gas is liberated from the cylinders as they empty.
    C. It is a safe practice to partially fill an empty cylinder from a full cylinder.
    D. It is useful for measuring low flows,

16. **The "second messenger," important in hormone action, is :**
    A. Adenyl cyclase
    B. Protein kinase
    C. 3', 5'-cyclic adenylic acid
    D. Adenosine 3'-5' monophosphate

17. **The "storage lesions" of whole blood with CPD solution include following except :**
    A. A decrease in 2, 3 -DPG
    B. A decrease in plasma hemoglobin level
    C. A decrease in red cell viability
    D. An increase in plasma bicarbonate

18. **Isoflurane has the following characteristics :**
    A. It has almost the same vapor pressure as methoxyflurane.
    B. It causes no respiratory depression.
    C. It has only limited biodegradation.
    D. It can produce bromism in very long procedures.

19. **Which of the following is essentially completely metabolized in humans :**
    A. d-Tubocurarine
    B. Atracurium
    C. Vecuronium
    D. None of the above

20. **Chlorpromazine is effective against following except:**
    A. Uremia-induced emesis
    B. Emesis due to gastrointestinal irritation
    C. Apomorphine-induced emesis
    D. Nausea due to vestibular stimulation

21. **Thiopental in clinical doses has a marked depressant effect on :**
    A. Liver function
    B. Hear rate
    C. Neuromuscular transmission
    D. Cerebral metabolism

22. **Shivering increases whole-body oxygen demand by :**
    A. 50%   B. 100%
    C. 150%   D. 250%

23. **Thiopental given intravenously to the parturient patient will appear in the cord blood in :**
    A. 30-60 seconds   B. 2 to 3 minutes
    C. 10 to 15 minutes   D. 15 to 20 minutes

24. **The anaesthetic considerations in patients with severe aortic insufficiency should include following except :**
    A. The avoidance of bradycardia.
    B. The avoidance of halothane or other agents likely to produce hypotension.
    C. The monitoring of pulmonary artery pressure.
    D. The avoidance of tachycardia.

25. **Following spinal anaesthesia the onset of headache in a patient ambulating after surgery is most common on the :**
    A. Day of operation
    B. First day after operation
    C. Second day after operation
    D. Fourth day after operation

26. **One-lung anaesthesia is mandatory in following except :**
    A. Bronchopulmonary lavage
    B. Bronchopulmonary fistula
    C. Pulmonary abscess
    D. Pneumonectomy for cancer

27. **The causes of pulmonary shunting include following except :**
    A. A severe diffusion block
    B. The bronchial circulation
    C. Atelectasis
    D. The Thebesian veins

28. **Halothane interacts with ketamine to produce following except :**
    A. ↓ CO   B. ↑ HR
    C. ↓ BP   D. None of the above

29. **Propofol has to be given with special caution in following except :**
    A. Epilepsy   B. Dyslipidaemia
    C. ↑ ICT   D. Asthma

30. **Onset of action of halothane is :**
    A. 30 sec   B. 3 mins
    C. 5 mins   D. 10 mins

31. **Duration of action of Vecuronium is —— min.**
    A. 5-10   B. 10-15
    C. 20-30   D. 45-60

Ans.	15. D	16. C	17. D	18. C	19. D	20. D	21. D	22. D	23. A	24. D
	25. B	26. D	27. D	28. B	29. D	30. C	31. C			

32. **Following are special precautions for Vecuron except :**
   A. Severe obesity
   B. Malignant hyperthermia
   C. Bronchospasm
   D. None of the above

33. **Following causes resistance to ketamine :**
   A. Ergometrine   B. Naltrexone
   C. d-TC   D. Alcohol

34. **Propofol dose has to be reduced with :**
   A. Methoxyflurane   B. Enflurane
   C. Isoflurane   D. Vecuronium

35. **Halothane causes the following :**
   A. ↓ Urine production   B. Polyurea
   C. Bronchoconstriction   D. Cough

36. **Which of the following when used with ketamine increases risk of seizures :**
   A. Aminophylline   B. d-TC
   C. Thyroxine   D. Oxytocin

37. **Blood brain equilibrium with propofol use is achieved in :**
   A. 15-30 sec   B. 30-60 sec
   C. 1-3 min   D. 3-5 min

38. **Vecuronium has increased effect with following except :**
   A. Lignocaine   B. Quinidine
   C. Verapamil   D. Theophylline

39. **Following decreases the effect of Vecuronium :**
   A. Tetracycline   B. Neostigmine
   C. Carbamazepine   D. Ganglion blocker

40. **In acute respiratory acidosis, the change in pH for each 20 mm Hg increase in $PaCO_2$ over 40 mm Hg will be :**
   A. 0.05   B. 0.075
   C. 0.10   D. 0.125

41. **A combination of low CPV and peripheral vasoconstriction is found in :**
   A. Barbiturate intoxication
   B. Fever
   C. Fluid loss
   D. Opiate intoxication

42. **The most important first step in the management of all shock states is :**
   A. The administration of vasopressors
   B. The use of positive inotropic drugs
   C. Effective beta-blockade
   D. Ensuring adequate intravascular volume

43. **The Apollo astronauts tolerated an F102, of 1.0 for 2 weeks without any complications. This was possible because the pressure in the Apollo capsule was :**
   A. 760 mm Hg   B. 380 mm Hg
   C. 260 mm Hg   D. 210 mm Hg

44. **The pressure exerted by 1 mm Hg equals how many cm H_2O:**
   A. 1.28   B. 1.32
   C. 1.34   D. 1.36

45. **The PaO_2 is lower than the PAO_2 even in normal lungs due to following except :**
   A. Normal "shunting"   B. Bronchial circulation
   C. Thebesian veins   D. Anatomic dead space

46. **In normal lungs in the upright position, the $PaCO_2$ in the apices is :**
   A. 28 mm Hg   B. 32 mm Hg
   C. 36 mm Hg   D. 42 mm Hg

47. **At the mitochondrial level, the PO_2 may be as low as :**
   A. 1 mm Hg   B. 2 mm Hg
   C. 3 mm Hg   D. 5 mm Hg

48. **How much time do the erythrocytes have in the resting human to accomplish pulmonary gas exchange:**
   A. 1 second   B. 2 seconds
   C. 3 seconds   D. 4 seconds

49. **The normal value for total peripheral resistance is :**
   A. 8,000 to 11,000 dynes.sec/cm⁵
   B. 50 to 150 dynes.sec/cm⁵
   C. 300 to 500 dynes.sec/cm⁵
   D. 900 to 1,500 dynes.sec/cm⁵

50. **Fentanyl induces muscle rigidity. The activity :**
   A. Is not reversible with naloxone.
   B. Is more common after the rapid administration of larger doses.
   C. Is responsive to succinylcholine but not to gallamine.
   D. Occurs because of fentanyl's action at the neuro-muscular junction.

51. **The normal dibucaine number is approximately :**
   A. 90 to 105   B. 70 to 85
   C. 55 to 65   D. 35 to 50

52. **Propofol may cause following except :**
   A. Ophthalmoplegia   B. Tremor
   C. Pain in injection   D. Cardiac arrythmias

53. **The duration of action of Pipercuronium is ——— times more than alcuronium.**
   A. 2-3   B. 3-4
   C. 5-6   D. 8-10

Ans.	32. D	33. D	34. C	35. A	36. A	37. C	38. D	39. C	40. C	41. C
	42. D	43. C	44. D	45. D	46. A	47. A	48. A	49. D	50. B	51. B
	52. D	53. B								

54. Following are special precautions for pipercuronium use except :
- A. Myaesthenia
- B. Hepatic Function impairment
- C. Severe obesity
- D. Malignant hyperthermia

55. If respiratory acidosis is chronic, the change in pH for each increase in 10 mm Hg in Pa CO_2 over 40 mm Hg will be ———— meq/L.
- A. 1.5
- B. 3.0
- C. 4.0
- D. 5.0

56. Meperidine reaches foetomaternal equilibrium in ———— min following I/V anaesthesia.
- A. 3
- B. 6
- C. 9
- D. 12

57. Best PEEP means :
- A. The higher the PaO_2, the better the tissue oxygenation.
- B. The highest level of PEEP that can be used safely is 10 mL H_2O.
- C. There is a level of PEEP that results in the best total O_2 transport of the blood, even though a higher PEEP may result in a higher PaO_2.
- D. The PEEP at which the PaO_2 is lowest.

58. The pregnant woman at term requires a dose of local anaesthetic for epidural anaesthesia that is :
- A. 15% more than the usual
- B. The same as usual
- C. 15% less than the usual
- D. 30% less than the usual

59. The average expected duration of action of tetracaine in spinal anesthesia is :
- A. 30 minutes
- B. 60 minutes
- C. 90 minutes
- D. 120 minutes

60. In an average 40-years-old man, an epidural injection of 20 mL of 2% lidocaine at L-2 would be expected to block how many segments.
- A. 8
- B. 12
- C. 16
- D. 20

61. If the $PaCO_2$ is 95 mm Hg and the patient is breathing room air, the PaO_2 cannot be more than :
- A. 20 mm Hg
- B. 30 mm Hg
- C. 40 mm Hg
- D. 50 mm Hg

62. If total circulatory arrest is required, the tympanic temperature must be about :
- A. 0° to 5°C
- B. 5° to 10°C
- C. 12° to 15°C
- D. 15° to 20°C

63. Provide other factors do not change, increasing the FIO2 to 0.3 should increase the PaO_2 by :
- A. 15 mm Hg
- B. 25 mm Hg
- C. 42 mm Hg
- D. 65 mm Hg

64. The indications for mechanical ventilation include all of the following except :
- A. PaO_2 less than 60 mm Hg with an F102 of 0.5.
- B. Vital capacity less than 15 mL/kg.
- C. pH less than 7.25 if this is due to hypercarbia.
- D. $PaCO_2$ of 50 mm Hg.

65. The dose of protamine administered following extra corporeal circulation must be :
- A. 1 mg/kg
- B. 1 mg for every 50 units of heparin remaining
- C. 1 mg for each unit of heparin given
- D. 1 mg for every 100 units of heparin remaining

66. During total bypass perfusion, mean arterial pressure should be maintained :
- A. Between 25 and 50 mm Hg
- B. Between 40 and 90 mm Hg
- C. Between 100 and 120 mm Hg
- D. Between 120 and 150 mm Hg

67. Flavoxate is used in :
- A. Renal colic
- B. Angina
- C. Headache
- D. BHP

68. Sodium Picosulphate is used in :
- A. Diarrhoea
- B. Constipation
- C. Intestinal obstruction
- D. GB colic

69. Bupivacaine may cause following except :
- A. Cardiac arrythmias
- B. Respiratory failure
- C. Hepatic dysfunction
- D. Nephrotic syndrome

70. Thiopentone is contraindicated in following except :
- A. Addison's disease
- B. Status asthmalcus
- C. Thyrotoxicosis
- D. Status asthmaticus

71. Duration of action of ketamine (I.V.) is :
- A. 30 sec. to 1 min
- B. 2-3 min
- C. 5-10 min
- D. 10-15 min

72. Nicorandil is :
- A. Antianginal
- B. Antibiotic
- C. Immunostimulant
- D. Antiarrythmic

73. Following are interactions of lignocaine except :
- A. Cimetidine — ↓ lidocaine clearance
- B. Propranolol— ↑ lidocaine levels
- C. Tocainide — ↑ adverse reactions
- D. Theophylline — effect blocked

Ans.	54. B	55. C	56. B	57. C	58. D	59. C	60. C	61. B	62. C	63. D
	64. D	65. D	66. B	67. A	68. B	69. D	70. C	71. C	72. A	73. D

74. In 4 hours period, maximum dose of bupivacaine is ——— mg.
    A. 50
    B. 100
    C. 150
    D. 250

75. Following are side effects of ketamine except :
    A. Tachycardia
    B. Nystagmus
    C. Epilepsy
    D. Bronchospasm

76. If there is 20% shunt, the percent inspired oxygen needed to restore normal PaO_2 is :
    A. 30
    B. 57
    C. 67
    D. 97

77. Chest wall compliance is ——— per cmH_2O.
    A. 0.11
    B. 0.21
    C. 0.31
    D. 0.41

78. If the PaCO2 is 95 mmHg and the patient is breathing room air, the PaO2 can not be more than ——— mmHg.
    A. 20
    B. 30
    C. 40
    D. 50

79. The name chloroform was given by :
    A. Von Liebig
    B. Guthrie
    C. Soubeiran
    D. J.B. Dumas

80. Blood take about ——— sec. to pass through capillaries.
    A. 0.5-1.0
    B. 1-2
    C. 3-4
    D. 5-6

81. Who first recorded the electric current that precedes muscular contraction of the heart :
    A. Von Liebig
    B. A.D. Waller
    C. William Harvey
    D. Soubeiran

82. Normal airways resistance of below ——— cm $H_2O/l/s$.
    A. 1
    B. 2.5
    C. 5.0
    D. 10.0

83. Halothane was sythesized by :
    A. W.G. Bigelow
    B. C.W. Suckling
    C. Macintosh
    D. Corssen

84. The normal metabolic cost of breathing is about ——— ml O2 per l/min of ventilation at rest.
    A. 0.5-1.0
    B. 1.0-1.5
    C. 2.5-3.0
    D. 3.0-3.5

85. The oil/water coefficient of Thiopentone is :
    A. 2.3
    B. 3.7
    C. 4.7
    D. 5.3

86. Following are effects of etomidate except :
    A. ↓ RR
    B. ↓ HR
    C. ↓ Cerebral blood flow
    D. ↓ Intraocular pressure

87. Resistance to propofol anaesthesia is countered by giving :
    A. Steroids
    B. Opioids
    C. 25% increase in dose
    D. 50% increase in dose

88. Thermoregulatory threshold (TRT) for propofol/ N_2O is :
    A. 31°C
    B. 33°C
    C. 34.5°
    D. 36°C

89. GA decreases responses to hypothermia by about :
    A. 1°C
    B. 2.5°C
    C. 5.0°C
    D. 7.5°C

90. Caffeine - halothane contracture test is used to screen a patient for :
    A. Hypotension
    B. Hypothermia
    C. Malignant hyperthermia
    D. Renal output failure

91. Post-operative shivering can be stopped by using the following except :
    A. Applying radiant heat to face or chest
    B. Pethidine
    C. Doxapram
    D. Atropine

92. GA raised the activation threshold for responses to hyperthermia by about ——— °C :
    A. 1
    B. 2
    C. 3
    D. 4

93. In freezing water, one survives ——— min naked.
    A. 2
    B. 5
    C. 10
    D. 30

94. There is an inverse relationship between plasma calcium and ——— interval.
    A. PR
    B. QRS
    C. QT
    D. R

95. An increase in pulmonary vascular resistance is caused by :
    A. Acetylcholine
    B. Adrenaline
    C. 5-HT
    D. Alveolar anoxia

96. In acute renal failure, the substance most likely to cause physiologic derangement is :
    A. Urea
    B. Potassium
    C. Creatinine
    D. The bicarbonate ion

97. A reduction in $PaCO_2$ from 40 to 20 mm Hg decreases cerebral blood flow by :
    A. 25%
    B. 30%
    C. 40%
    D. 50%

Ans.	74. C	75. D	76. B	77. B	78. B	79. D	80. B	81. B	82. B	83. B
	84. A	85. C	86. B	87. B, D	88. B	89. B	90. C	91. D	92. A	93. C
	94. C	95. A	96. B	97. D						

98. The resting tidal volume to vital capacity ratio should be :
    A. 1 : 50   B. 1 : 20
    C. 1 : 10   D. 1 : 5

99. What portion of the tidal volume is normally represented by dead space:
    A. 2%   B. 10%
    C. 35%   D. 40%

100. The helium dilution method measures :
    A. Tidal volume
    B. Total lung volume
    C. Dead space
    D. Functional residual capacity

101. Most common untoward effect of the thiazides is :
    A. Hypernatremia   B. Hypokalemia
    C. Hyperchloremia   D. Hypocalcemia

102. Blood stored for 14 days contains normal amounts of :
    A. Factor-V   B. Factor-VIII
    C. Prothrombin   D. Platelets

103. In the resting humanbeings, the time taken by the erythrocytes to accomplish pulmonary gas exchange is —— seconds.
    A. 0.5   B. 1.0
    C. 2   D. 4

104. Dextran-70 may produce coagulation difficulties if given in doses exceeding ——— ml :
    A. 500   B. 1000
    C. 2000   D. 3000

105. Which of the following drugs potentiates the effect of Warfarin sodium :
    A. Paracetamol   B. Barbiturates
    C. Rifampicin   D. Cimetidine

106. Ketamine should not be used in patient with except :
    A. Penetrating eye injuries
    B. SLE
    C. Psychiatric disorders
    D. Raised intracranial pressure

107. The cardiovascular complication of oxytocin therapy is :
    A. Hypertension   B. Bradycardia
    C. ST-T changes   D. All of the above

108. In hypotensive anaesthesia, the mean arterial pressure must be maintained above —— mm Hg.
    A. 20   B. 30
    C. 40   D. 60

109. Isolation of morphine from opium was first done by ——— in 1806 :
    A. Baron Larrey   B. J.A.C. charles
    C. Thomas Beddoes   D. F.W.A. Serturner

110. Normal coronary blood flow at rest is ——% of cardiac output.
    A. 1   B. 2
    C. 5   D. 7.5

111. During total bypass perfusion, mean arterial pressure should be maintained between —— mmHg.
    A. 20-40   B. 40-90
    C. 90-120   D. 120-150

112. Helmut Weese is famous for introducing :
    A. Methoxyflurane   B. Muscle relaxation
    C. I/V anaesthesia   D. Local anaesthesia

113. In Bowen's syndrome, there is sensitivity to :
    A. Halothane
    B. Muscle relaxants
    C. Dissociative anaesthetics
    D. Sedoanalgia

114. In elderly and short obese, blood volume is ——% less than normal adult.
    A. 5   B. 10
    C. 20   D. 30

115. Provided other factors do not change, increasing the FIO2 to 0.3 should increase the PaO_2 by —— mm Hg.
    A. 20   B. 35
    C. 45   D. 65

116. Curare was first described by :
    A. S.L. Auenbrugger   B. Stephen Hales
    C. P.M. Angherius   D. J.A.C. Charles

117. Following is useful in Armadillo's disease :
    A. Regional blockade   B. Sleep
    C. Phenytoin   D. Atropine

118. If total circulatory arrest is required, the tympanic temperature must be about ——— °C.
    A. 0-5   B. 8-10
    C. 12-15   D. 18-20

119. Following are features of Albright Butler syndrome except :
    A. Hypokalemia   B. Acidosis
    C. Hypercalcemia   D. Hypomagnesemia

120. Propofol prolongs the half life of :
    A. Neostigmine   B. Thiopentone
    C. Atropine   D. Alfentanil

Ans.	98. C	99. C	100. D	101. B	102. C	103. B	104. B	105. D	106. B	107. C
	108. C	109. D	110. C	111. B	112. C	113. B	114. B	115. D	116. C	117. C
	118. C	119. D	120. D							

121. Duration of action of Sufentanil is ——min.
   A. 1-5
   B. 5-10
   C. 30-60
   D. 60-90

122. Ketamine anaesthesia is partially reversed by :
   A. Atropine
   B. Physiostigmine
   C. Droperidol
   D. Naloxone

123. Suxamethonium interacts with following except :
   A. Erythromycin
   B. Lithium
   C. Aprotinin
   D. Ecothiopate eye drops

124. Azepexole acts on —— receptors.
   A. Alpha-1 adrenergic
   B. Alpha-2 adrenergic
   C. 5-HT
   D. Noradrinergic

125. The curve which the lungs follow during inflation is different from that during deflation. This behaviour is called :
   A. Dalton's law
   B. Hysteresis
   C. Gas-pressure difference
   D. Haldane effect

126. Gasser's classification is used to classify :
   A. Inhalant anaesthetics
   B. Anaesthetic equipments
   C. Depth of anaesthesia
   D. Types of nerve fibres

127. Half life of Succinylated gelation (Gelofusine) is about —— hours.
   A. 2
   B. 4
   C. 8
   D. 12

128. Goldman's index of cardiac risk in non-cardiac procedures give maximum score to :
   A. MI in preceding 6 months
   B. Rhythm other than PAT
   C. 3rd heart sound
   D. Age > 70 years

129. Hagen-Poiseuille formula includes all of the following except :
   A. Pressure gradient across tube
   B. Radius of tube
   C. Viscosity of fluid
   D. Density of fluid

130. Hamburger shift is related to :
   A. H^+
   B. Cl^-
   C. Na^+
   D. Ca^{++}

131. Campbell and Howell method is used to measure:
   A. Arterial pO_2
   B. Arterial pCO_2
   C. pH
   D. Viscosity

132. Main problem faced in Chadiak-Higashi syndrome is:
   A. Difficult intubation
   B. Recurrent infections
   C. Hypoglycemia
   D. Respiratory depression

133. "Crash induction" is mainly used to decrease risk of:
   A. Hypotension
   B. Aspiration
   C. Cardiac arrythmia
   D. Vagal shock

134. The air exchange area of the lung consists of the following except :
   A. Alveolar sacs
   B. Respiratory bronchioles
   C. Alveolar ducts
   D. Lobular bronchioles

135. A major advantage of high-frequency oscillatory ventilation is :
   A. Decreased cost
   B. Decreased inspiratory pressure
   C. No need to intubate
   D. No need to humidify the oxygen or air used

136. Pressure exerted by 1 mm Hg equals —— cmH_2O.
   A. 1.28
   B. 1.30
   C. 1.34
   D. 1.36

137. In normal lungs in the upright position the $PaCO_2$ in the apices is ——mmHg :
   A. 28
   B. 33
   C. 35
   D. 38

138. At the mitochondrial level, the PO_2 may be as low as —— mm Hg.
   A. 0.5
   B. 1.0
   C. 2.5
   D. 5.0

139. Which of the following is structurally related to meperidine :
   A. Metoclopramide
   B. Methadone
   C. Dextromoramide
   D. Fentanyl

140. Scopolamine delirium can be reversed by :
   A. Diazepam
   B. Physostigmine
   C. Thiopental
   D. None of the above

141. Henry's law relates to following most important factor of gas :
   A. Amount of gas
   B. Partial pressure
   C. Concentration
   D. Temperature

142. Normal Hufner's constant is —— ml/g.
   A. 1.12
   B. 1.39
   C. 1.51
   D. 1.85

143. 'Hofmann degradation' is seen in :
   A. Pipecuronium
   B. Atracuranium
   C. Suxamethonium
   D. Vecuronium

Ans.	121. C	122. D	123. A	124. B	125. B	126. D	127. B	128. C	129. D	130. B
	131. B	132. B	133. B	134. D	135. B	136. D	137. A	138. B	139. D	140. B
	141. B	142. B	143. B							

144. **Name of "Magill" is also used for a :**
    A. Face mask   B. Laryngeal mask
    C. Intubating forceps   D. Stilette

145. **Hagen-Poiseuille formula applies to :**
    A. Newtonian fluids
    B. Non-Newtonian fluids
    C. Blood only
    D. All of the above

146. **Smith-Lemli-Opitz syndrome is characterized by all except:**
    A. Micrognathia   B. Mental retardation
    C. Thymic hyperplasia   D. Difficult intubation

147. **Polysplenia is often associated with:**
    A. T-cell dysfunction
    B. Congenital heart disease
    C. Diabetes insipidus
    D. Adrenal failure

148. **Alfentanil has——times potency to that of fentanyl.**
    A. 1/4   B. 1/3
    C. 1/2   D. 2

149. **Brodsky test is used to determine patency of:**
    A. Pulmonary artery   B. IVC
    C. Ulnar artery   D. Long saphenous veins

150. **Brown and Miller effect is seen due to sudden reversal of:**
    A. Hypercapnia   B. Hypoxaemia
    C. Hypotension   D. Hypothermia

Ans.   144. C   145. A   146. C   147. B   148. A   149. C   150. A

ANAESTHESIA

References Quoted

S.No.	Books
1.	Lee's **Synopsis of Anaesthesia**. ELBS, London
2.	**Goodman Gilman's The Pharmacological Basis of Therapeutics.** McGraw Hill, NewYork
3.	Bhatia's **Quick Medical Text Review, Anaesthesia.** CBS Publishers & Distributors Pvt. Ltd., Delhi, 2010

Unforgetable Supplement

Bhatia's **Quick Medical Text Review Series** (Quick revision of all the subjects in short time. No need to underline the books (read important points). CBS Publishers & Distributors Pvt. Ltd., Delhi.

SHORT TEXTBOOK OF PSYCHIATRY
(Aids to Psychiatry)

About this Book (New Edition)

- This new book is specificially written for easy grasping of Psychiatry in a clearent, pointwise, simple and easy understandable language and is exlusively based on the **examination oriented** pattern.

- A list of headings important for **Undergraduate** and **Postgraduate examinations** are given at the starting

- Various **Question Papers** of Psychiatry from previous years of many national undergraduate examinations have been added at the end of book.

- **Multiple Choice Questions (MCQ's)**, asked on various Undergraduate and Postgraduate Examinations have been added at the end of book

- Each chapter ends with **important points** enlisted in abox

- A section on the general principles of Psychiatry with a special emphasis on the Historical aspects (indian/Western), **Symptomatology** and Psychiatric Examination has been included.

- An updated section on Psychiatric Treatments including newer advances and list of all **Psychotropic Drugs** in alphabetically order (according to trade names) have been added.

- Important detailed chapters on Indian Psychiatry (Contributions of Indian Psychiatrists, Epidemiology of various disorders, National Mental Health Programme of India, Forensic Psychiatry, Indian culture bound syndromes etc).

- An important list of appendices include **Psychiatric Glossary,** list of **Psychological Tests, Psychiatric Side effects of Medical Drugs** etc.

- Useful book for various Medical Competitive and Undergraduate Examination; Civil Services Examinations

- Edited by : **Dr. M.S. Bhatia** (M.D., Dip. W.P.A.) an experienced teacher and examiner, associated with editing of many popular books on undergraduate and Postgraduate Examinations.

CBS Publishers & Distributors Pvt. Ltd.
NEW DELHI ● BANGALORE ● PUNE ● CHENNAI ● COCHIN (INDIA)